Those Micro Preemie Eyes

A memoir

In memory of Tanya Lansky

Copyright © 2022 Maria Zak and Sasha Zak

All rights reserved. No part of this book may be reproduced in any form by an electronic or mechanical means, including information storage and retrieval systems, without permission in writing from the publisher, or with proper citations.

The events in this book have been set down to the best of the author's ability, although some names of individuals and towns have been changed to protect the privacy of individuals.

Illustrations copyright © 2022 Maria Zak
Photography copyright © 2022 Maria Zak

ISBN- 978-1-7386383-6-9 : Paperback (Black White Version)
ISBN: 979-8-8298038-5-8 : Paperback (Colour Version)
ISBN: 978-1-7386383-7-6 : Hardcover (Back White Version)
ISBN: 979-8-8298352-3-1 : Hardcover (Colour Version)
ISBN: 978-1-7386383-2-1 : Ebook

Karacter Media
www.karactermedia.com
Hamilton, Ontario, Canada

Contents

Chapter One - Pregnancy In Trouble   1
*Living with low fluid * Hospital stay * Empathy * Coping*

Week 20	The Warm Drip	3
	My Future Leaks Through	5
	From Curtain Cell to Curtain Call	10
Week 21	At Home Bed Rest	15
Week 22	The Faded Map of Viability	17
	The Chicken Bucket	21
Week 23	Torture Across the Curtain	22
Week 24	The Count Down Begins	24
	I See Baby!	26

Chapter Two - The NICU   31
*Viability * Pumping * Procedures*

Week 25	Smile	33
	Wide Awake	37
	No Celebration	39
	The Touch	42
	Papa Moment	44
	Pumps	46
	I Find My Wings	48
	Preparing To Leave	49
	Viability Talk	50
	Nothing is Promised	53
	Home	54
Week 26	His Name	55
	Eyes	55
	Back to School	56
	The Cry	58
	Milestone Photos	59
	First Skin To Skin Cuddle	60
Week 27	Breathing Tube and Blood Transfusion	62
	Kilo Club	64

	PICC Line Removal	64
	Procedures	65
	Daddy's First Cuddle	66
Week 28	Routine	67

Chapter Three - The Waiting Game   71
*Mental health * Life outside of hospital * Celebrations*

Week 29	First Newborn Portraits	73
	First Parent Moment	74
	Pump Activism Is Born	76
	Geoff	81
	The Machinery	84
	C PAP Milestone	86
Week 30	Future Is NOW	88
	My Pump Routine	89
	Getting Sick	90
Week 31	Thanksgiving	91
	What Is In My NICU Bag	92
Week 32	Would- Be Born Today	93
	Eye Test Result	94
	New Activities	95
	Bad News About His Lungs	96
Week 33	Donation Time	98
	Onesie Milestone	101
	Halloween Costumes	101
Week 34	Two Month Anniversary	103
	Legally Alive	103
	Not Compromising Expectations	104
Week 35	Fat	105
	Another Vacancy	106
Week 36	Crib Milestone	108
	NICU Monologues	110
Week 37	Feeding Schedule Milestone	111
Week 38	Self Care	112
	Not A Social Worker, A Demon	113

Week 39	No C PAP Milestone	115
Week 40	Due Date	118

Chapter Four - The Last Battle — 123
*Level 2 Ward * Breastfeeding * Broken system*

	Level 2	125
	Christmas and New Year	128
4 Months	Bunk Room	130
	Mother Vs Malerie	132
	The Luxury	139
	Crying Over Spilled Milk	144
	They Win	146
	The Last Place.	150
5 Months		150
	Newborn Photography	152
	Like Home.	154
6 Months		156
	The Face with No Tubes	156
	Care By Parent Room	157

Chapter Five - Life After Hospital — 163
*Written by Sasha Zak * Early intervention*

First Six Months	165
At Home	166
First Two Years	167
Physical and Cognitive	171
Together	171
Feeding Issues	171
Five Years Old	172

Chapter Six - Today — 173

About Authors	179
The Campaign	181
Index	183

Chapter One
Pregnancy In Trouble

miscarriage not a swear word

Week 20

The Warm Drip

A few weeks ago ...
I raise my head in shock. The next assignment is worth 40 percent of our whole grade. That is almost half! And we have a week to complete it. I fly my hand up and ask why it is so high for such a short amount of time to complete.

"What if I have a miscarriage then?" A mixture of uncomfortable mutters and giggles ripple behind me.

"I might have one you know? One in four women have them."

My classmates knew that I was pregnant long before that sacred three months mark, when, it's usually kept a secret. I have spent three very intensive and intimate years with them, in this Masters of Social Work course. I told them if I have a miscarriage, they would find out anyways because it would be impossible to keep secret. I might as we let them know ahead of time that I was pregnant. In the meanwhile the goofy performer in me wants to change society one tiny activist statement at a time. Today's theme is the desensitization of miscarriage. However in just a few weeks I shall find out that after 20 weeks it's called an early pre-term delivery.

***

All these formulas and numbers that are in my Research Methods course. I am not a numbers person. Yawn. If I close my eyes will the professor notice? I'll just look down and pretend to be writing notes.

Today...

I am making tea at my desk. It is a meditative process. I bring out my fresh lemon and ginger and cut them into little nuggets. Am I allowed to bring a sharp knife to class? Next I add loose tea and dry berries to create a red warm fruit fusion in my teapot and wait for it to cool. It's a warm August day and here I'm with my warm tea, sweating. I shift around on my wet sticky chair and pour the lovely goodness ever so slowly into my cup. This is also part of the process, the pour. It's not only romantic but also helps distract me from my nausea that still persists even though I am entering my sixth month now.

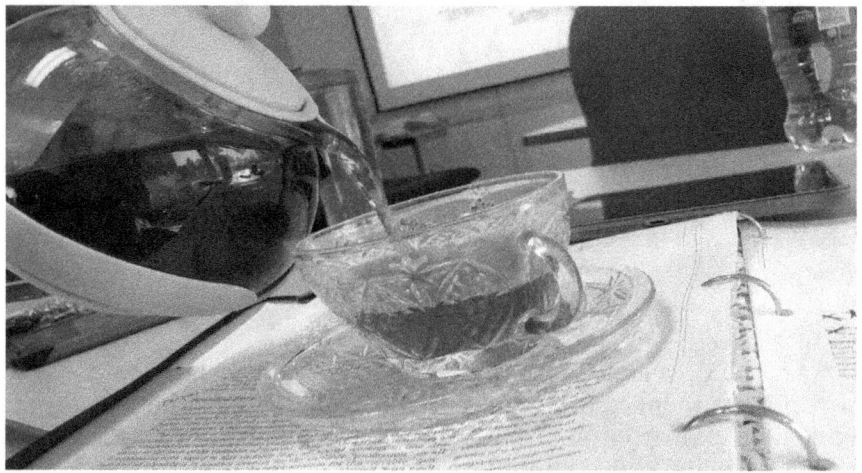

Did I just feel something extra? I put my hand under me to examine if the seat is wet. Dry. I return to my tea. However, it keeps feeling extra moist and is now a bit higher, somewhere between my legs. No! Please no. I've been here before. Please. Anyone with a period will know this anxiety on a regular day, but when you are pregnant, it's not an embarrassment that's on your mind. I raise myself slowly with my back to the wall and look to see if my chair is wet. No it's fine. My clothes seems dry as well. In the bathroom the revelation is the colour bright red. Take a breath, dial my midwife. She tells me to monitor it, to watch out for clots and how much bleeding is happening. She then recommends that I go home to rest. I return to my classmates with a fake business as usual smile, but it doesn't work. They see my pale face with the fear in my wide eyes, and reciprocate with an empathetic inquisition. My confession tells them that I was worried about my pregnancy for the last couple of weeks and even visited the ER last week. They insist that I go home and promise to finish the work for me. It's a strict program and I haven't missed a day. But now I have to go home early for the first time. It's a long ride home as the warm blood continues to drip like that cherry chromed tea.

My Future Leaks Through

The following day I wake up with a startle at discovering that my bed is soaked with water. I have drenched my sheets right to the mattress. There are also blood clumps there. I try to investigate what I am seeing, heart beating hard. Water and splatters of blood. The horror, the anger and the fear. I'm taking deep breaths to calm down and not send any negative energy to the baby. I feel him kicking happily. He loves his morning exercises.

> *I felt his movements very early, at 14 weeks. He would poke me most often when I was on the bus clenching my hands on plastic bags in case of a random throw-up attack. I would smile at my companion. He liked to toss around in my belly at night and always wanted to lie on the side where I preferred to lie. I would let him choose a side while I lay facing the other way. He was so playful, and we were already best friends.*

As a towel collects my fluids, I hunt the internet for my symptoms. I see fossils of people before me. Run, they shout.
After I bled for two weeks, I lost the baby.
       .. Light bleeding is fine.
  cramps ...   death ....   miscarriage
don't worry!   yes worry!

The summary of the internet oracle is that I'm in huge trouble. I'm like that woman who bled for two weeks. During this pregnancy I had two close people lose their babies. One lost hers at the end of her first trimester, the other was a beauty who died two weeks after birth. I admit that I had pregnancy guilt. My pregnancy was hard. I had to quit working because my midwife told me to choose school or work because both were too overwhelming. I entered the world of living on the poverty line pretty quickly. Ideas like starting a mortgage one day or getting a car were all postponed. I also lost my ability to get maternity pay. But I was blissfully pregnant and the happiest person. Not because pregnancy completed me, but rather because I have fulfilled all my dreams and now ready to add to my family. My career was great. My body achieved all my acrobatic dreams. All I had left now is my Masters degree and a baby. Bliss! Yet guilt.

I find my emergency cash and take a taxi to the nearest hospital emergency in Yorkton. The driver chats to me as I pretend that I'm fine and not worrying about staining his car seat through my many layers of toilet paper in my underwear. I try to imitate his calm demeanour as he talks to me, while contemplating whether or not to call l my husband Geoff. Do I worry about my family?

Once at the hospital, I stand in the registration line. Water breaks through the barrier and starts to trickle down my leg. I'm scared to look up. If someone noticed I'm too ashamed to have my eyes meet with their judgments. The far away spot on the floor between the giant tiles is where I stare. Registration doesn't process me but instead sends me straight to their maternity ward. Maternity is on the other side of this indoor city. Pushing my stubby legs and heavy belly forward as fast as I can, without running, I rush to wherever I think is the most direct way to safety.

'Please don't notice me,' I think as I pass helpful security personnel trying to see if I need help.

The statue of Mother Mary greets me as I enter. She is supposed to be comforting standing there all maternal, but not this time Mary. Sorry. At least I think I'm in the right place. I wipe the water blur out of my eyes and through the choke of my nasal tears I explain the water breaking. The admin tells me that I haven't registered with them, and I technically should not have come there. *If you ever can hear eyes rolling through someone's tone of her voice.* I tell them that their ER sent me here. I went to their own emergency section! Like any person with a problem would.

"Do I return to the general emergency then? What should I do?" I shift my legs as my barrier gets heavy and sags down my thighs.

"Fine, we'll do what we can, take a seat," the cold voice returns.

I've never felt like such a burden. The need to apologize for my problem. My midwife's hospital is two hours and three buses rides away. As anyone else would do with any ER situation, I came to my nearest hospital. It had not occurred to me that I had to be registered anywhere to be treated. Maybe the final birth, but not for emergency purposes. They place me on a bed, and a doctor examines me. He says he'll be back shortly with the results. My two options are that this is a urine infection which can be treated. Or my water broke, and it's the beginning of the end.

This binary answer shall determine my entire life going forward.

As fast as that doctor shuts the door, a nurse enters to tell me to please leave, this bed is reserved for someone later today who *has* registered. They show me the waiting room and ask me to wait for the doctor's return. I fear sitting upwards and wonder if I should be lying down to slow the leaking. There's nowhere to lie down. The chairs have arm rails. I try to take slow breaths to calm myself and my baby, who has no idea of the magnitude of result I am anxious to hear.

Minutes of impatience turn to hours, and this time line is now a blur. After ten hours of musical chairs with my wet face and shorts, it's almost midnight. I try another go at begging for the doctor. The nurses' short returns are that he's at another birth and cannot sign me out or diagnosis me. They are too busy to care for me. I'm not their patient. My shame in asking these overworked nurses for special attention shuts me up as I nod sweetly and limp back to my wet chair. I'm not angry at them. I do my best at using a soft voice, not to stress them anymore. After all, who am I to them? A nagging nobody who should not have had a leaking problem when they are in a busy maternity ward. My path back shows a glimpse of my former bed so urgently needed for someone else. It's still empty. I suppose it's someone who will use it after surgery. How lucky they are. I want to have surgery and have a baby on that bed too.

Geoff is new in his job, so we decide to keep him there for his long shift. He just got a great animation position and it's our only income. We can't lose this job. Geoff needs to stay there.

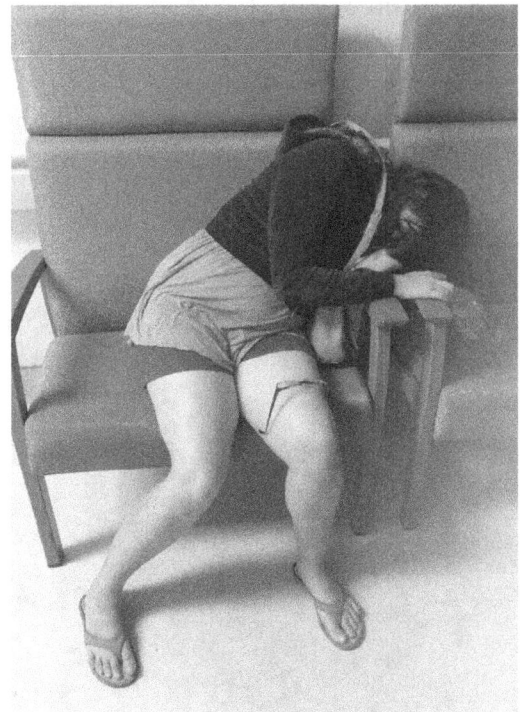

My sister, Sasha arrives instead from Hamtown, a ways away, to support me. We contemplate suing if something happens to me that might be prevented. This musing perhaps is my best distraction of the night. But whom to sue? It's not this doctor's fault. He is alone here. It's not the nurses' fault that they don't have the authority to diagnose me. Do we sue the government for under-funding hospitals? How? Regardless of it all, it kept us occupied for several hours.

Eventually, it's already the next day shining smugly on the clock on my phone. I tell them that either my baby is dying or it's a thing that will fix itself, but I feel safer waiting it out with bed rest at home. They give me a form to sign to take the responsibility off the hospital and throw out all my suing aspirations. Reluctantly, I start to drag myself home. On my way out I tell the nurses that all the seats here are wet and that they should sanitize them. As I walk away, I see their big eyes on me as though they have noticed me for the first time.

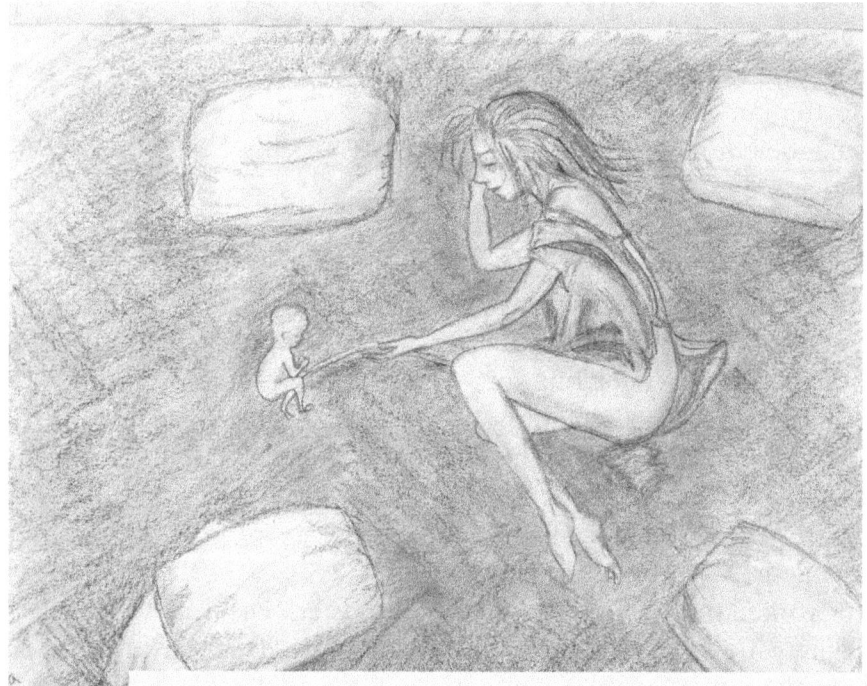

I don't remember where I was when I got the call, or what I was doing. But now I am running. I run through the corridors, past the nice security guard , then the Mother Mary. Until I run into her huddled over a chair arm in the quiet empty waiting area of the maternity ward. In my arms I have clothes for overnight and snacks. I assumed the decent next step was offer medical help. Possibly over night. But unfortunately this isn't the reality. I arrived as soon as I could. My husband is waiting outside in the car. She sat on wet chairs for ten hours. I take the photo of her crouching over. I need to capture this injustice in case someone will listen. Instead it only makes me cry. Sorry Maria, I wish we could trade places.

Sasha's perspective

The following day with my midwife's advice, I go to the hospital where she registered me in Thornton. I make that sleepy journey over three buses. Baby doesn't kick with this one. We are both sitting silently. I study the frivolity of each passenger and envy their innocence as they get on with grocery bags.

At this hospital, they approve me with urgency. My midwife is my ticket to help. The doctor examines me with cold tools. By now, I'm bleeding heavily. I'm not scared, not worried, nothing. I have no energy to feel anything anymore. They change me into a hospital robe, and I get a bed with all the bells and whistles of an IV and a hospital tag—such a contrast to last night where I was invisible.

My midwife comes in. I ask her if this is the beginning of the end, she looks away with a barely visible nod. Her eyes blink wildly, probably suppressing tears. I do my quirky 'I'm good' routine with inspirational poster phrases about climbing mountains and something about meaning. It doesn't matter what I'm saying. I'm on auto pilot again. I just want my midwife to feel better. In truth, I am scared. The mist of death is hovering over me.

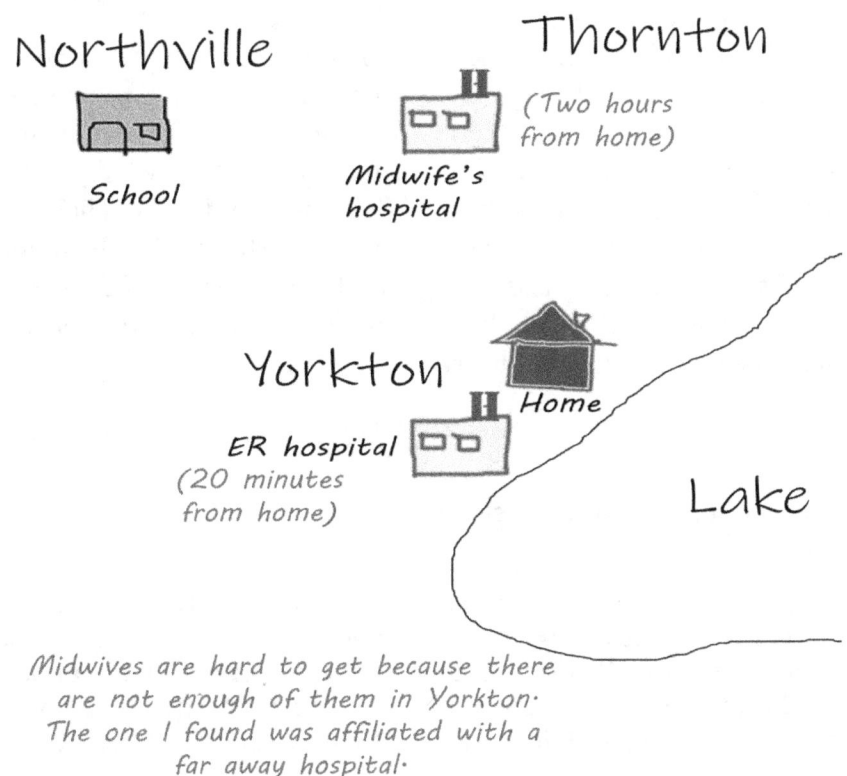

Midwives are hard to get because there are not enough of them in Yorkton. The one I found was affiliated with a far away hospital.

From Curtain Cell to Curtain Call

I spend a week in this curtained cell. If this was a dream, I'm now awake. I have to say it out loud. I am losing my baby. This is what it is like. I'm now that person. Practical thoughts enter the mind. Do I use up the name Elyot, that I like, on this baby whom I shall lose, or do I save it for the next? Do I tell people now as it's happening, or do I give them a summary later? Do I allow myself to feel this or run from it? And how big is this clot?

My room has two beds. I'm closer to the entrance door. Every visitor to the other patient walks through my badly curtained area. They smile and apologize for disturbing me. Then I see their smiles fade as they look at me. I think my face tells them everything.

Later I look at myself in the mirror to see what others see. I look sad. Not a hint of anger, nor fear, just a sunken face with no hope. There is no poetics there, no complexity of emotions, just sadness. I have never seen this face on me. This is not me. I feel disassociated with the lady looking back. There's no person there, just darkness. And if these visitors can see it within the glaze of my eyes, then so shall my family.

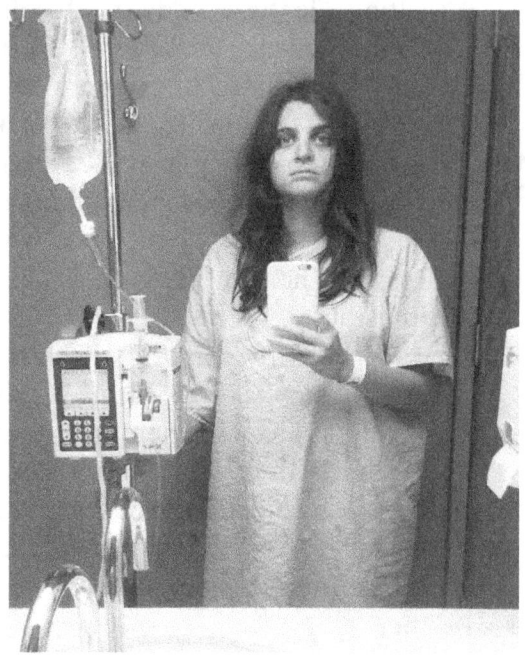

If I suffer, so shall they. I need to show them that I'm brave so that they can be courageous. I have to care for more than myself and my baby. There are Geoff and my family. They know me to be cheerful. So for them, that is what I shall remain. I decide to become strong. This experience won't defeat me.

 Maria Zak updated her status.
August 18, 2016

Update: I don't like to share personal stuff like this on FB but it's a thing that people shall notice anyways. So here goes : I'm in hospital in critical condition for my baby. We don't know if baby will survive. It's been a hard month. A day at a time. But instead of feeling sorry for me please be inspired by how strong and deep I am. This time too shall pass.

I look down at my vibrating phone. There must be dozens of missed calls by now. Everyone worrying. Before I call them back, I need to set the tone. I take out my phone and start to practice smiling. No, it's still sad looking. Let's try another. Though there is nothing natural about the poses, they do have a contagious aspect to them. They start to make me laugh. It works. I am distracted enough and start to have fun. My silent giggles move me into the next theme of my life. I'm a bloody inspiration! Eager fingers on the phone send these to my anxious family who are glad to see me in high spirits. I can hear them through their words in texts. They pick up in energy and positivity. Now I can phone them back. Once they have been taken care of, I make my social media posts using these photos. I tell my family and friends that no matter what happens, I'm still me, and nothing will break me. I'm going to show everyone how to find new life when amid death!

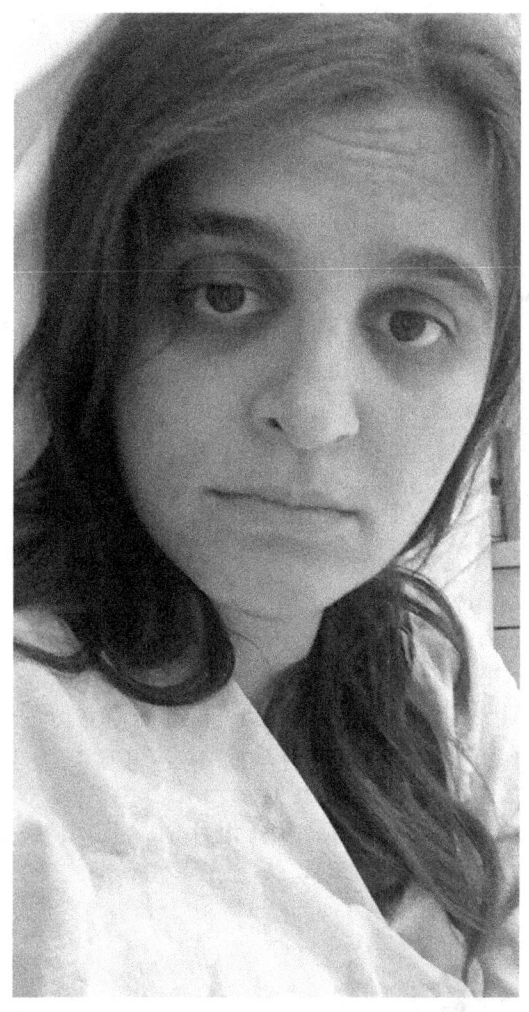

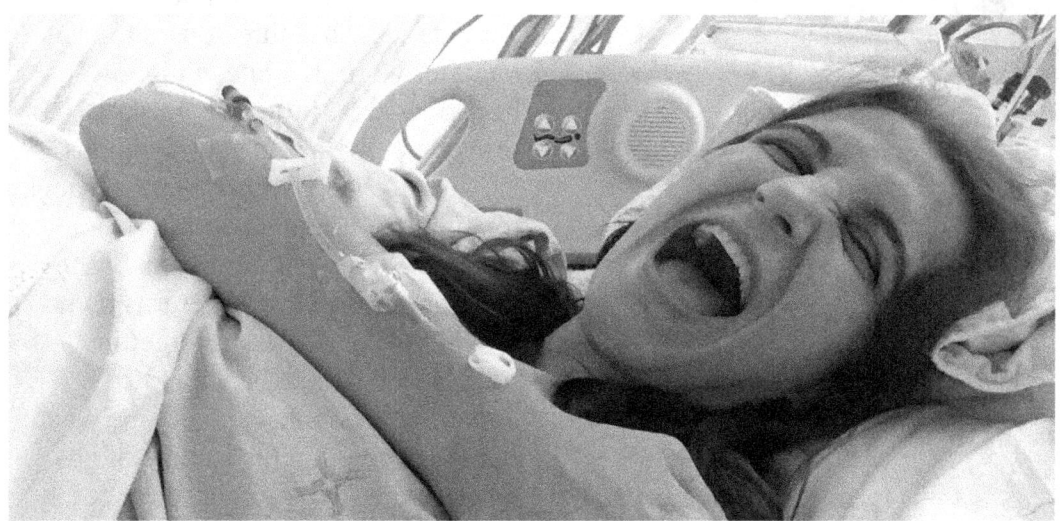

The first night here, you realize that at night you get no sleep. They come in several times to check on you. They do a full vitals check and ask about the bleeding. Each time they turn on the lights and irritate the under-slept over-cried eyes. When they are not waking me up, the drip empties sounds loudly. I wake up in a panic, wondering what's wrong with me, what's this sound? The nurses are in no rush to come and fix it. It just continues until they have time to appear and turn it off. In the morning, I wait for the doctor to come, but he doesn't. No one with the title of doctor does. The nurses can't tell me anything. I watch them continue their rounds with no rush and assume that I'm not urgent to them. That thought relaxes me back to my moving mountains slogans. But after not getting much sleep since last night it's hard to get into that mind set.

Sentimentality aside, I still have a lot of assignments to complete for class. I have quizzes and group projects left. After a couple of days here, I begin to find new energy to get some work done.

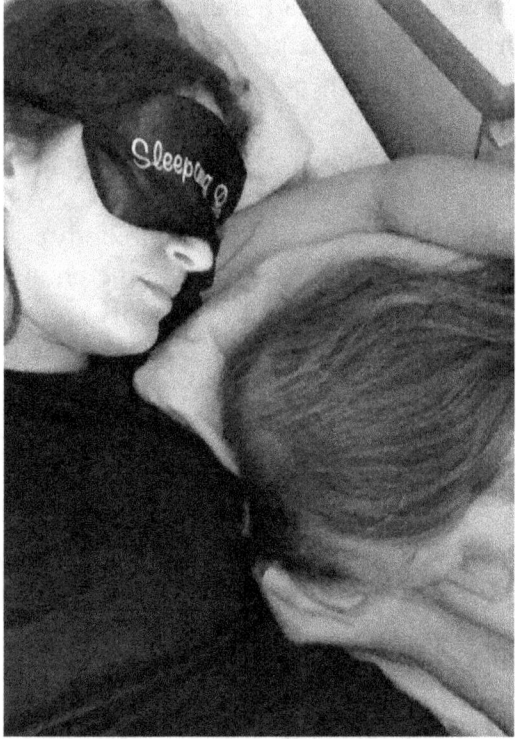

This hospital is far from home, and Geoff takes those three buses to visit me after work. It's late at night when he arrives with little time to stay. He brings me my laptop and textbooks. He doesn't have the privilege of shock to numb the mind. He's experiencing it all raw. Also visiting me makes his work suffer because he returns home too late. We can't risk him getting fired, so we decide he should stay home. Now no one can visit me where I am. I'm stuck in the middle of nowhere in my tight corner of the room.

Their ultrasounds show nothing wrong. It's a puzzle. Years later, they will tell me I had an infection that led to this fluid loss, but today they don't know why this is happening. Today they want to make sure that I am safe from any severe infection or blood loss that can be life-threatening. They can't save a baby at 20 weeks, just me. Yet today, no one appears acting urgently.

They seem to be waiting for this thing to pass. Fear turns to boredom. I try to spend this time with writing and film editing. Anything to waste time on the computer. It's a small room and feels more like a giant elevator than a bedroom with nothing visible apart from the curtains surrounding me.

I spend my days wondering what's outside the window. Eventually, I get a glimpse while the bed by the window is empty. It's the view of another grey hospital wall and a parking lot. I'm not missing anything. I chuckle to myself at how disappointing that view is. I do prefer being closer to the toilet on my side anyway.

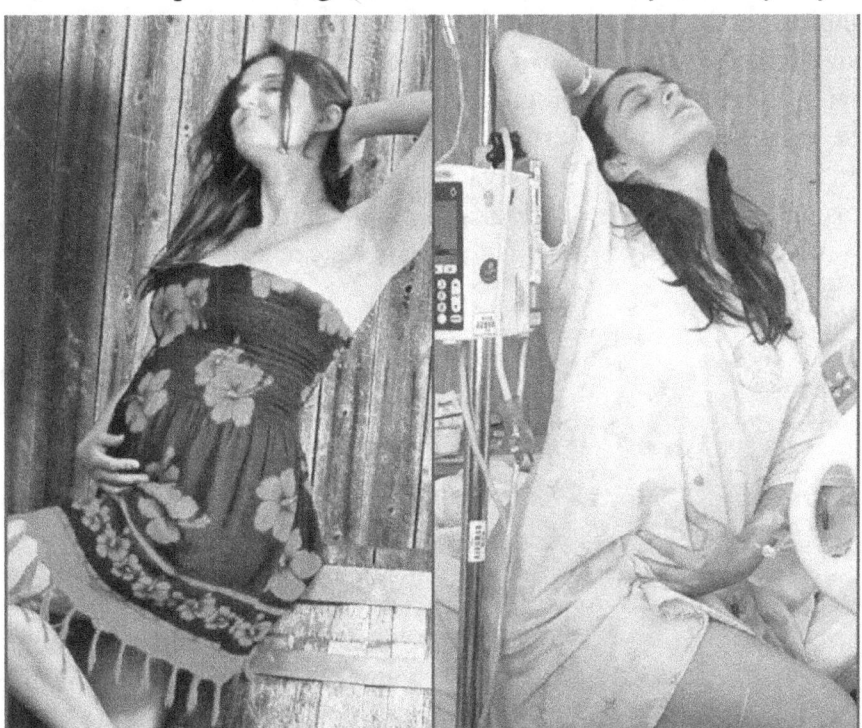

This photo is my way of saying goodbye. The first photo was taken at four months. I was waiting to be seven months pregnant for my next photos.

Baby, if you go, my spirit shall follow you.

As they continue their vitals checks each night and force me awake, I lie there in the silence listening to the cries of mothers in the vast corridors as their contractions come. It is raw, shameless and free-spirited. I envy the innocence of that pain. In the mornings, I hear choruses of happy families striding in like it's their home. They carry gendered balloons and tiny flowers with stuffed animals that one can buy at the store downstairs. Their joy is loud and imposing. Their energy irritates me as I limp to the toilet to check on the blood and take pictures of my clots to show the nurse later. They give me massive pads to collect the blood and water. Every time I change one, I have to save it to weigh it to track the bleeding. The nurse also checks my underwear with her vitals checks during the day. Just opens up the bed sheets and looks inside. Whatever modesty I once had does not exist here.

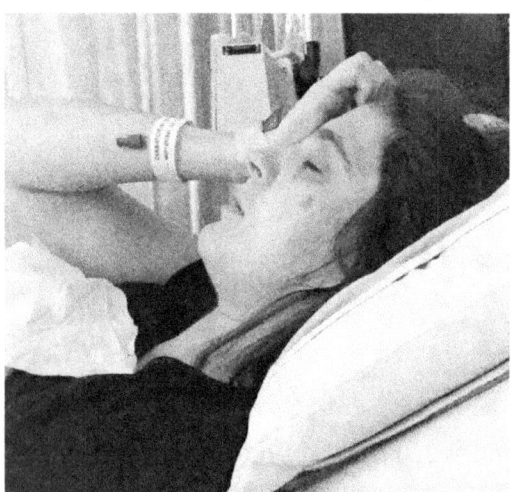

Meanwhile, my chamber changes patients. A lady on the other side of the curtain is 23 weeks pregnant. Something to do with a short cervix that needs to be sewn. She gets 'the talk.' She needs a translator to understand the doctor. He tries to simplify his speech. I hear the stress in his voice. He says to her, 'if your baby is born this week, it only has a 50 percent chance of surviving; however, if you last till next week Monday when it's 24 weeks, it increases to three quarters." I don't hear her talk, so I wonder how much of the message she is getting. I cry myself to sleep, thinking of her and wondering if she understands her situation. She does eventually last till Monday and goes home because her risk level improves. I'm only in my 20th week. My chances are so bleak as reality starts to set in. I yearn for 24. But it seems impossible at this point.

***

It's not a hospital for extreme cases. Usually they are discharged to another hospital or home. You never find out what happens to anyone unless they came here for a full-term birth. Several chamber sisters have come and gone. They left me with me their secrets that probably their own friends don't even know. Their stories burn me. They are all in the middle of the waiting game. At this point, I am unaware that I was sharing a room with the future me's.

Week 21

At Home Bed Rest

After a week in the hospital, the bleeding stops, they find no reason to keep me. My experience here is summarized with a doctor shrugging his shoulders as he examines my chart. They send me home on strict bed rest with no explanation for what happened.

It's good to be in a home again, at my in-law's place in Hamtown. Here they can take care of me. No more living through others' joys and sorrows. No more beeping noises or temperature checks to keep me awake. My sleep is my own again. However, once home, it all returns that same night. It happens in a pattern of transparent water, then pink, then red, then just water again. The wetness that started with a crawl is now in a hurry. I leak as I change positions on the couch. It accompanies me when I stand up to go to the washroom. At night it wakes me up like a negative thought. It just continues to leak. I record the bleeding to share with my midwife. The hospital discharged me, so I am confused about what to think. Am I back in trouble again?

What's happening?

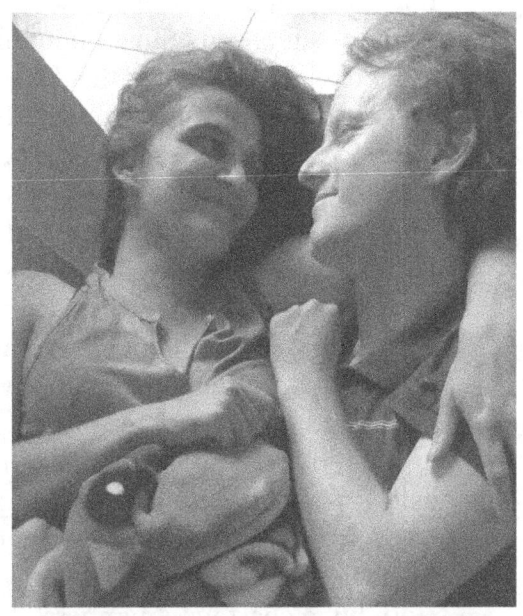

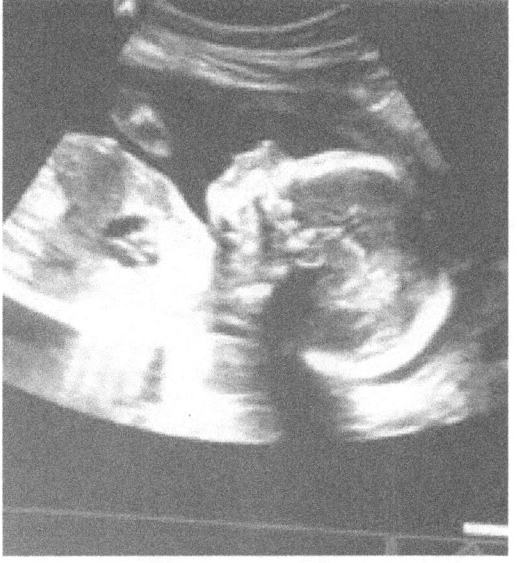

After another week at home, I get an ultrasound. It's one of those internal ones. A slimy and cold mechanical probe detective will find out what's happening. I know it's bad news because the technician mutters something under his breath. His non-words tell me more than whatever it is that he's saying. I have to go home and find out from my midwife what this secret is. Time moves slowly as she receives the results the next day when I get the call. We finally find out what's wrong. It's something they call low fluid. From the day I was discharged till today, I lost most of my fluid. It took a week. That stuff before was just a rehearsal; now we are here. I'm losing the water that's trying to keep my baby alive. My voice is calm, but my eyes gather up lakes as I complete my conversation. When I hang up, I wail. I wail an ugly cry. She does her last advocacy and gets me registered into a local Hamtown hospital close to most of my extended family. With one phone call, I'm exchanged from a caring midwife I know on first name basis, to a hospital team of strangers who introduce themselves to me as resident doctors of today. I'm no longer a person with a story but a chart with numbers. I arrive at the Hamtown hospital triage. More ultrasounds, blood tests and 'the talks' follow. It's my third hospital if you don't count the various emergencies before the pages of this book.

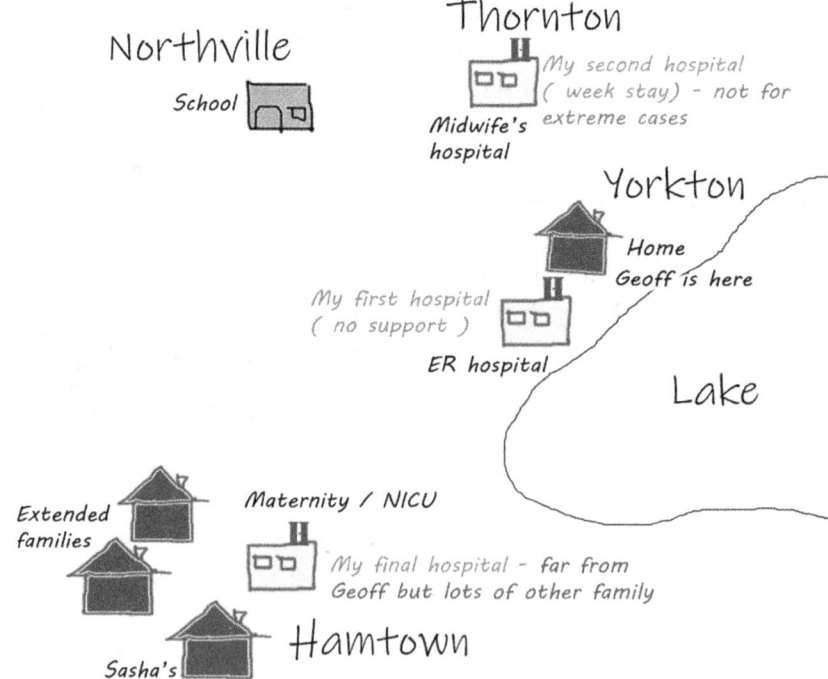

Week 22

The Faded Map of Viability

The doctor tells me that I have a slim chance to make it to 32 weeks. At this point I will be induced because a baby with my low fluid cannot go longer than that. They tell me a medium case scenario is 28 weeks. That is very premature, but on the safer side to have a good quality of life. However, a baby as low as 24 weeks would have to undergo intense therapies and treatments. The internet will tell me all the risks we could `face being born so early. Survival would not be the only thing to be of concern, but so will be the rest of his life.

The last case scenario is if he's born before 24 weeks. They will not save him. There will be no life. He is currently very small for a baby at 21 week gestation, and with low fluid may not grow much. Babies need to get bigger to be saved. He's also breech with little chance of turning. That makes the high probability of him or the umbilical cord to fall out and cause brain damage. They warn me often to press the emergency button if I feel something coming and to stay in bed with only minimal exceptions to go to the toilet or shower, nothing else. And meanwhile, watch out for lime-coloured discharge because that's another end. I hope you reach your destination.

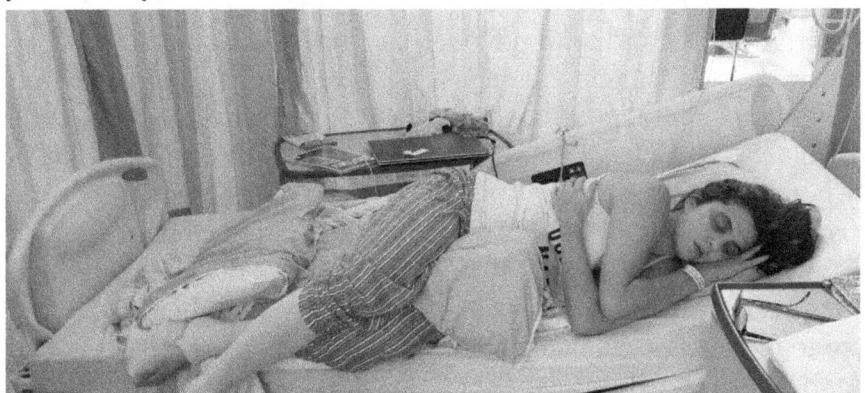

Boom boom, boom boom, boom boom. The cold tool searches for his heart rate. He's in a different place each time. He hates this tool and moves away from the microphone against my belly. With him goes the boom boom. But the nurse always finds his boom boom..

Keep drumming away little one. Please!

Experiencing nature move by as if it doesn't care about me, unaware of me, makes me feel left out. It's hurrying when I want the clock to stop. To figure out what I'm feeling right now. I drown in the thought of how big the future seems.

The guilt.

I feel remorse towards my unborn baby, healthy inside but might lose his life just because the placenta ruptured. I'm so sorry that you are ready for a beautiful long life that…. might not be. I decide that I no longer like the number 24. After reading all the risks to the child when they are born 24 -26 weeks. I no longer crave that number. *You are so healthy now, so playful in my tummy, and you might face significant setbacks if born so early.*
I negotiate in my mind which disability is worse on his quality of life. Which would hinder friendships, or accessibility, which are expensive. Will we need to move to somewhere with no stairs? Can I afford to move out somewhere else? I bargain among them. Sometimes I shut it all down because my future doesn't have you in it.

The ugly hope.

There is hope that I might last here till week 28 or more! That's when I feel time as a physical being. It's so big and so long. Like a road that leads into the dark. A night highway when on a road trip. Those empty fields below the naked sky. It's too big to comprehend. I feel so overwhelmed. I need to disappear from it, but how? It's in my brain! There is no 'off' button.

The bereavement.

I have already come to terms with the fact that this baby is going to die. I'm already planning out my life without him and how I shall deal with it. I rehearse in my head what I will say to people. I dread ahead of time all the pity that will come my way.

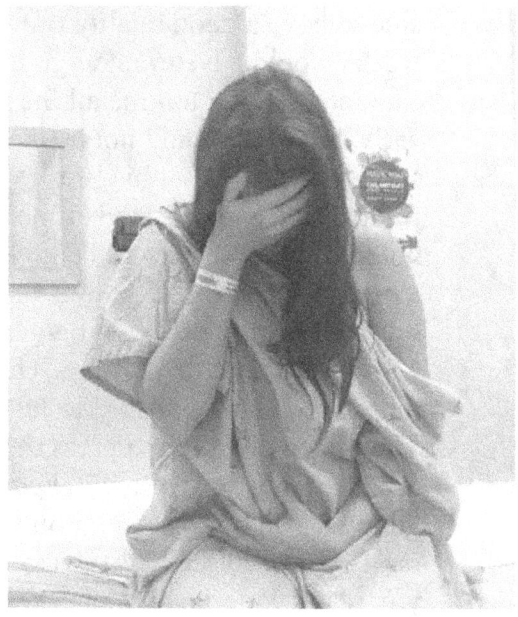

The loneliness.

There's an unexplained emptiness that keeps growing in me. The more I hide from my emotions, the emptier the vessel I become. I fear overhearing something happening to my ward mates. I lose my energy to feeling their pain. I have nothing left for myself. I'm hidden from this world that does know my secret. No Geoff. He's too far. No kisses to the forehead, no warmth of a living partner worrying alongside me. I miss him. Nights are darkness I have never known before. All is quiet, so quiet that it screams.

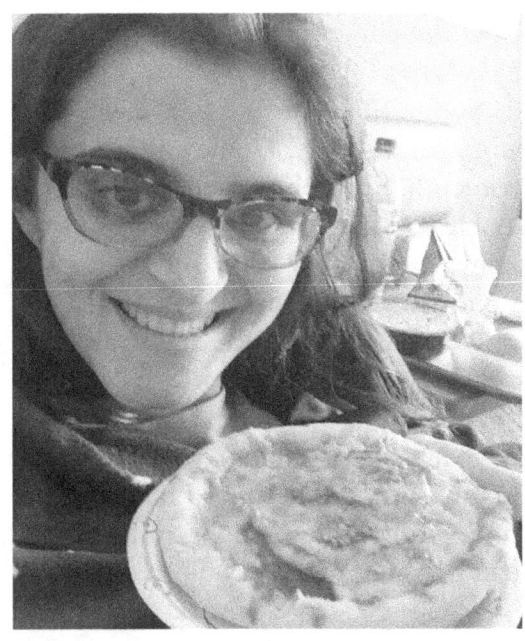

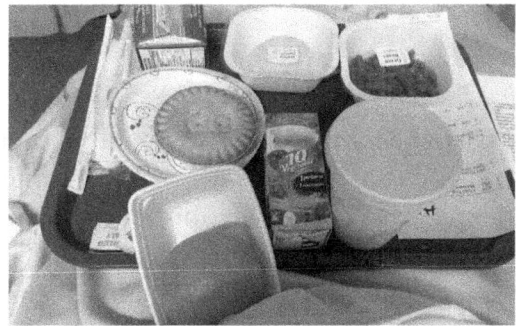

For entertainment, I watch Star Trek Voyager on an over-priced internet. I play chess with myself. I learn how to draw digitally on my tablet and continue to work on my writing. I share the password for my internet with some people. Most of them are here for a few days.

Meanwhile, as days turn into weeks, I become obsessed with my next meal. Patients who have extended stays get a special menu. I am self-conscious about my weight and try to pace myself with the pizzas. I enjoy their little pies. I order healthy food for the baby as much as I can. The coffee tastes like a powder mix, but I take pleasure in the process of sipping on the tiny Styrofoam cup. I save the desserts for Geoff when he comes. Sasha also often brings me healthy food from outside. Sometimes the kitchen messes up my order and gives me a generic meal that I didn't order. In those moments, I cry because it was nutrition taken from the baby. An obvious overreaction I know. I'm obsessed with feeding him because he is producing the amniotic fluid that I am leaking daily. In effect he is the one keeping himself from harm.

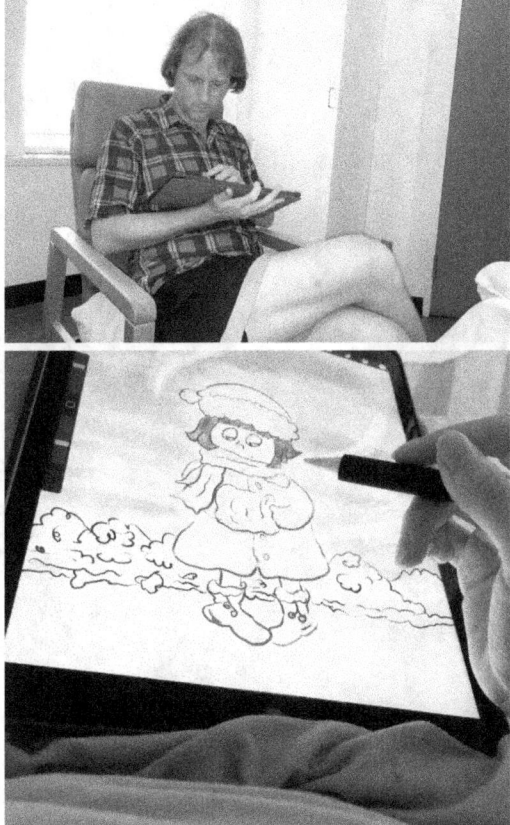

I try to get any possible essential nutrients for Maria's baby. Some stuff Maria doesn't want to eat so I shove them into her mouth. Spinach was one of those things. Also I read D is for bones. Definitely have to pack some protein for growth, and iron. I heard great things about sweet potatoes, I throw those in. Omega fatty acids for brain, this is a major one too. Throw in a bunch of nuts in the mix. Those are pricey, I'll deal with that later. I make smoothies with all the super foods I can obtain: ginger, onion, garlic, greens, berries, lemon. Its chunky and disgusting. Sorry Maria, just chug it. I figure out later to mix these in with tasty smoothies to kill the taste. A strawberry banana smoothie to mask the taste of garlic. Beets? Yes I probably add them in too, sorry. Sometimes I buy store made yummy drinks or pricey cold press drinks from coffee shops. Guilt has me spending. I also buy her cute pyjamas and try to arrange her hub so that it is cozy.

Sasha's perspective

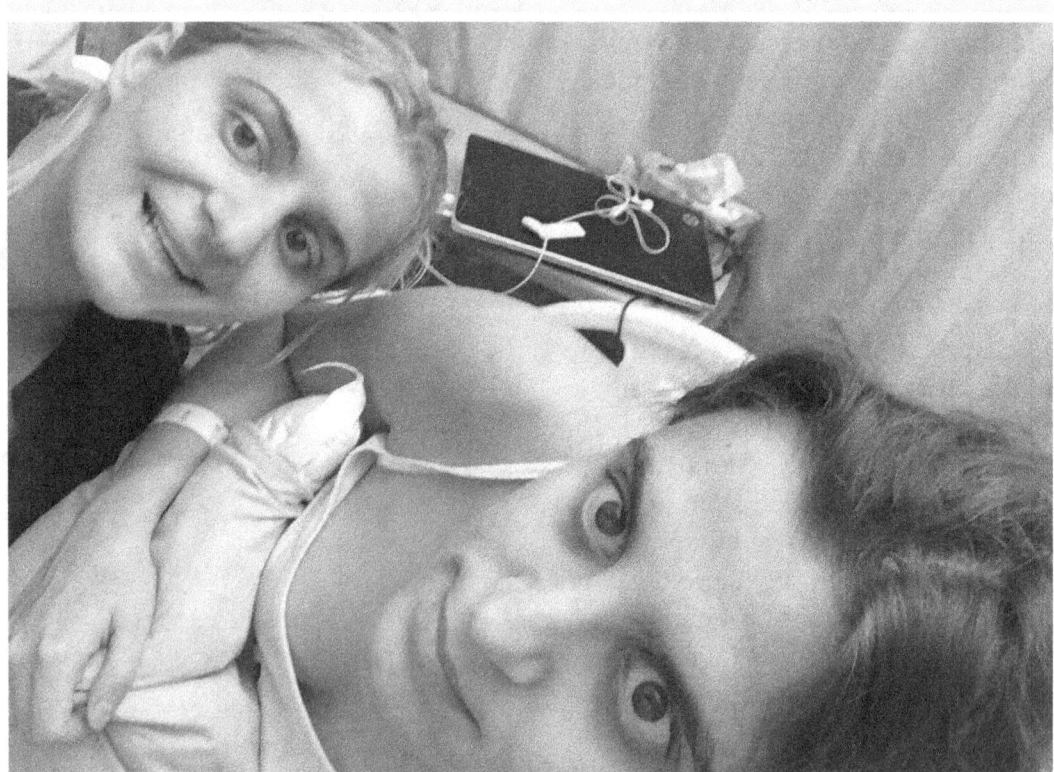

White Chicken Bucket

Everyone here loves chicken. Those chickens arrive in a white bucket. It's not a big deal. Maybe not worth mentioning here, but just a detail I noticed from my first days here. I even saw it displayed at night. They love chicken here!

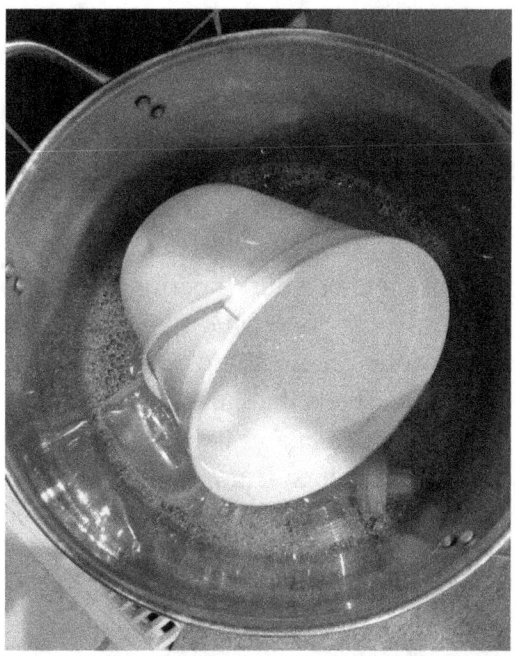

Some mothers would also get a sales lady coming in trying to sell them something. Did she bring them the chicken? It seems like the same people who talk to her have them. She is energetic and keeps saying phrases like 'you can do this,' 'you're amazing.' I wonder who that lady is and what is she selling? Is she selling private rooms in the hospital or an insurance plan? It feels wrong to sell anything in a hospital. All I know is that she comes to those who just gave birth. I decide that if she comes my way, I won't talk to her until I have family present. I have social anxiety and have trouble saying no.

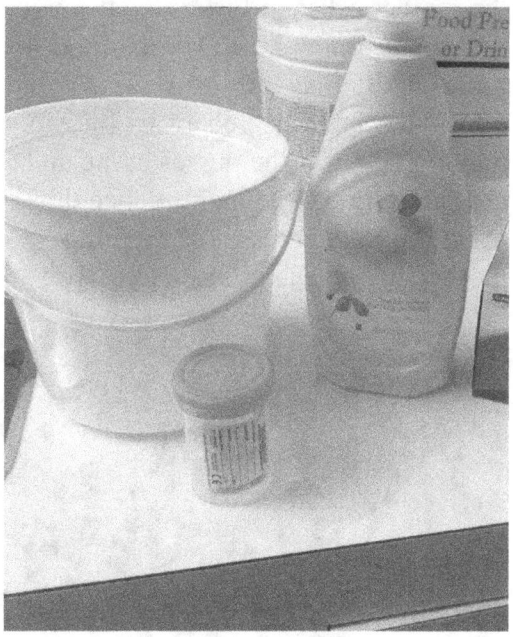

Later I learn that this is a lactation consultant, and she is selling them a lifestyle like no other, hope. She's talking to mothers at the lowest point of their lives and trying to uplift them. This ward is unusual where many parents have troubled pregnancies, so she brings her best cheery voice. She also brings chicken buckets. These buckets are containers for pump parts for breast milk for parents who cannot nurse their babies. It also doubles as a washing container in this germ-ridden hospital.

There was never any chicken.

Week 23

Torture Across the Curtains

Private rooms are for rich people only. Unless you can pay or have insurance, you have to share the space. The hospital can turn this room into two rooms, but they keep it as a four-bedroom anyways. The financial class system dictates your experience here. Several weeks here, and I hear everything around me. I share a room with three other beds that keep changing patients. Once again, I witness people's darkest moments. But now it's three stories all happening simultaneously. These people who, like me, are hidden from the outside world and are alone with their problems. I hear all the mothers' discomfort going through this stuffy room air as they toss and turn. Finally they tell the nurse it's that time. They are wheeled away. Later that night, I hear the nurses come and congratulate them. One sentence they often say to the premature birthing mothers is 'at least it's not so early'.

I later learn that they mean 28 weeks. None of them scream as they did at the previous hospital. None of them has regular births. Everyone here is in an emergency. The only sound they utter are soft cries into their pillows at night. One of them gave birth to twins and was unable to see them.

Another mother of a 27-weeker is begging to stay at the hospital longer to be closer to the NICU, the Neonatal Intensive Care Unit, that keeps premature or sick babies. Another one keeps phoning the NICU because her full-term baby suddenly needs a C PAP to breathe. She is scared. I often put in earphones to drown out other people's experiences around me. I absorb them, and they overtake me. Their experiences frighten me. Each one gives birth while here. I hear symptoms. I worry for each child. I fear for the twins just born. I worry every time they can't find a heartbeat somewhere. This place isn't for someone with even the tiniest compassion towards others.

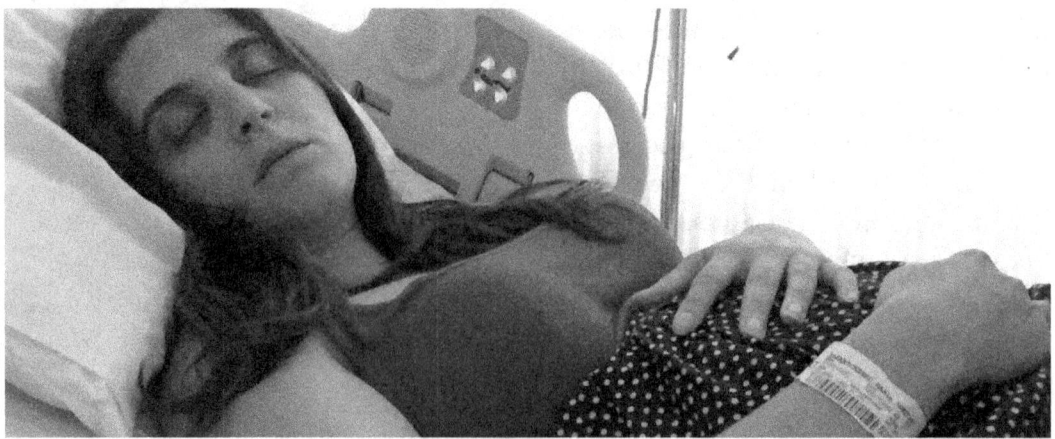

This part of my experience has produced the most stress and trauma as I go forward in life. It's torture by empathy. I feel their contractions. I feel their boredom. I feel their milk not coming in and the crying that always follows. I also feel the worry in the nurses' eyes, their maternal frustration when a mother gives up and stops pumping to rest and sleep for the night.

Another mode of torture here is sleep deprivation. Almost every night, the nurses bring a new patient. No one is quiet. The hustle and bustle of each new bed bringing in its first night of 24-hour vitals checks that wake them up, as well as, the bystanders sharing the room. There's no concern that people are sleeping. They are busy saving lives.

Also I'm bed-bound. I envy many of these patients who are allowed to go out for walks. Their babies are not breech and have no risk of falling out randomly. They have friends over and go out to eat in the cafeteria. The most I'm allowed is to walk to the toilet, or occasionally, the shower. I watch them return with their cake or pudding as they kiss each other goodbye for the night. Instead I make a friend here from my bed. She is going through the same low fluid as me. We become close. I share art supplies with her. So she, too, can be distracted with sketching. I become attached to her baby as I listen to their daily checkups and heartbeats; they sound like fast horses galloping.

I know everything about that baby and include it in my prayers.

I pray for everyone here. There isn't a single prayer for myself only. I want everyone to do well. I'm not religious, but praying has become a ritual here. I experience her losing her baby on the floor. That worst-case scenario I told you about. The baby falling out. It happens to her. There she is now crying out, "my baby!" The hustle-bustle of nurses rushing in. I don't know whose emergency button brought those nurses in but it's instant. Then it's silent. I cry into the pillow, and my body shakes uncontrollably. My friend just lost her baby. I will never hear its horse gallops ever again. Both are now gone without warning. A baby that can fit into the palm of a hand. Now gone.

***

They bring in Malerie, the social worker. She listens. She can't do anything for me but to listen. We talk of mindfulness – I have my art, and television shows to keep me occupied. We speak about depression. I tell her that I appear to be doing well according to The Edinburgh Postnatal Depression Scale (EPDS). Being a social worker myself, I have already assessed myself. She has nothing to tell me. She asks if I have something to say to her; I reply, "not at the moment." All I asked for was a semi-private room but I can't afford one. I don't need any counseling. She leaves me her card, and this talk is done.

Week 24

The Count Down Begins

Today I drag myself out of bed to brush my teeth and feel my belly. It feels like it doubled. I look in the mirror, and for the first time since my water broke, I look somewhat pregnant. What I will find out later after his birth is that he had a huge growth spurt. At this point, I am worried about his size because they told me he is small and might not grow. I hear the nurses tell parents that doctors can't save babies if they are too small. This has been my big worry. My friend who just lost her baby at 25 weeks, her baby was too small. I understand the consequences of a small size. And yet, he grew to my surprise.

An ultrasound tells them my cervix is getting short. I know at this point that I won't make it week 26. We celebrated each week's milestone with a cupcake; now I cancel it because I see no use. My leaking stopped. I wonder if the rupture has closed or if there is no more fluid left. They counsel me about different options of the Cesarean Section and when they would use each option.

Elyot is breech and with low fluid will not turn around to face down, so he will not be born without surgery. They tell me if he is born in the next few weeks, it will be a classical cut, a type of more invasive surgery. If he is born vaginally, he is at a considerable risk of an umbilical born injury. Then we discuss all that can happen if he is born super premature and all of our intervention options. They give me a precautionary lung steroid injection so that when he is born, he has this extra support for breathing.

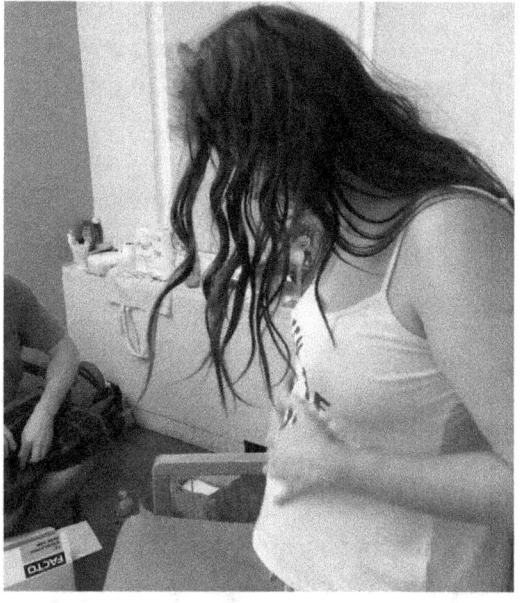

Morning of the big day: I run in to drop off any healthy snacks I could grab. I drop them off on my way to work. It is my obsession in my efforts to try save the baby. I return first thing after work with more snacks. I am tired after my demanding job, but Maria looks worse. She is huddled to comfort herself, as if sleeping, but she isn't. She can't find comfort. She tells me to go home because she has no energy for conversation. I can't leave her like this. I stay. My husband joins. The three of us sit together in silence.

Sasha's perspective

We start daily stress tests to get a record of his heart rate. If they suspect stress, they will take him out. I try to calm him with soothing music before we go there to save him from being taken out. Then back in the ward, I energize him with apple juice for the vitals checks and to get my daily kick count scores. It's a balancing game of keeping his heart at the right pace. I meditate to keep myself positive.

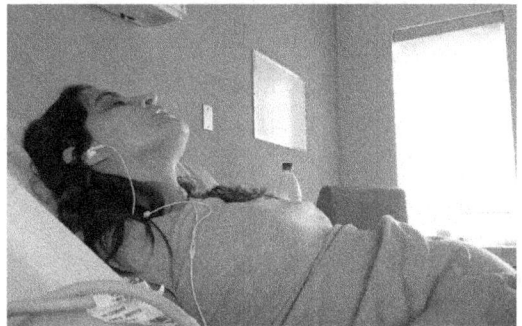

I keep thinking of what I heard at that ultrasound meeting- short cervix. No doctor has spoken to me about this. I know my days are numbered. Geoff is in denial and is convinced that I can make it to 32 weeks. I have no energy for his positivity. I can't relate to it and it tires me out. He keeps reading me statistics. He doesn't understand what a short cervix is. I'm exhausted from explaining. Mama calls from Boston many times a day over video chat. She wishes she was here to support me. I need her here. We don't even talk. We just sit together in silence and that's enough. My sister starts to stay with me longer. She falls asleep on the chair. She has a sense that my days are numbered and is afraid to leave me alone.

My baby doesn't share my sleeping positions with me anymore. He still kicks and nudges but he no longer moves around like he used to. There's no space to move with low fluid. I imagine him like a fish in shallow water. In reality he is surrounded by the fluid but a thin layer. But I imagine it like he's sitting in a puddle.

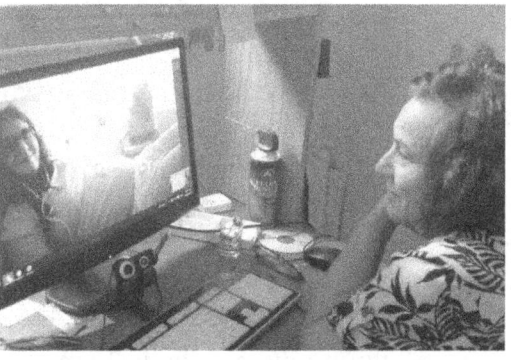

Maria doesn't do a great job hiding her fears, we all see it. Our mother who is far away develops a depression from this event. She cries herself to sleep every night. No one tells Maria this. She is right that this was not just her and the baby in this. We all are feeling it together. Meanwhile, I am working on their immigration applications to bring there here. Now we need our family together more the ever before.   *Sasha's perspective*

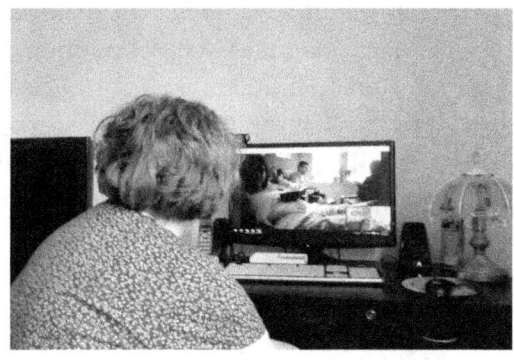

I See Baby!

I start to get a sore back and cannot sleep. Then on Thursday evening, I get what I think are tiny contractions. Pain isn't the accurate word for it, but a deep intense discomfort where no position is comfortable. I set a timer. At first, they are 15 minutes apart, but they become three or four minutes from each other quickly. Geoff is on the phone counseling me and trying to calm me. Sasha is here with me and refuses to go home in case something happens.

My nurse rushes me to triage to monitor me. Sasha follows. They try to avoid internal exams because it leads to infections, but this nurse makes an exception. What happens next stops my heart. She freezes and says, "I see baby!". Everyone in the room stiffens and begins to communicate urgency with their eyes. I find my sister sitting behind me in my peripheral. I don't look directly at her but send my whole energy towards her direction.

"We're losing Elyot, and it's okay. I am at peace." I tell her and I think I even mean it. I am at peace in this moment. Mostly I want my sister to be okay. She is pale when I finally glimpse her. I know that she is looking at me, but it seems more like looking through me, into that place where my fears, my future, and my innocence are all dying. I am numb and genuinely accepting the situation. Sasha is no longer playing along with false hope. She is sitting there looking cold. No smile. Her performance is gone. She has forgotten that her audience is still in front of her on the hospital bed. I reach my hand out and give her a small pat. She is experiencing her twin sister suffering and saying goodbye to her future.

One staff says a C section cannot be done. Too late. Another interjects that we have no moment to spare, it's time for surgery. I start to brace myself for bad. Maria seems so calm. Did she hear what they said? Staff is running crashing into each, but she is still. I watch the doctor announce that they are preparing for surgery. Maria's hand that I am holding firmly on my lap is pulled away as they surround her to place her and roll her away. I tuck into the corner as far as a can to get out of their way. Suddenly I am alone in here. With everyone gone I stand in silence.

Sasha's perspective

I notice her glasses in my tight hand that I am holding and her phone on the chair. I pick them up and her sweater that I brought in case if she got cold. The shock to my system as I remember Geoff. Outside my husband and mother in-law are already waiting. They recall later that I walked towards them with without blinking, torturing them with my extended silence. Right now all that I can muster up is a shoulder shrug while I approach them. It is at this point that I remember that Maria told me that its okay. " We're losing Elyot and its okay." It all rolls back to me now. I think I blocked her out when I was trying to figure out the staff. "She'll be okay! She'll be very very okay!" I turn to them with a smile. She has this!"

No time to save him?

More doctors rush into the room, and each one sees something new. This doctor sees a foot. Another person comes in to confirm, and I hear the words "umbilical cord". I have minutes left and might not make it to surgery in time. If he comes out now, there are few chances of saving him because of his umbilical cord. They turn to me with a long speech. I cannot hear anything. I just see their eyes trying to communicate something. I interrupt and ask them, "are you asking for consent for surgery? YES! Anything!" They put me on my side, roll me onto another bed and urgently rush me into the surgery room. Sasha and everything disappear. It all turns into a thick mist where only portions of events are visible to me. I try not to breath in case that movement will push Elyot out. I try to remain still. Not to twitch. My breathing is more like howling in fear. I am moaning loudly. I don't care what they think of me. I imagine how much of him has come out already and the brain damage that it's causing. Time has stopped to such a crawl that I have very detailed thoughts. As the anesthesiologists look for the perfect spot to give me an epidural, another nurse wraps her body around mine... Shh shhh. She rubs my shoulder with one hand and squeezes my hand softly with the other. Shhhhhh They turn me back around. Put a cover sheet to separate my face from the rest of the surgery. Are they cutting me while I am awake? Elyot's foot is out and on its way is the horrendous umbilical cord. I don't want to have consciousness while my son is perishing. I was wrong! I'm not calm about this!

I don't want to lose my baby. I ask them why they are not putting me fully asleep. I beg them to put me under. I have no more energy, so my exclamations are in loud whispers. They tell me it's better this way, and I'd suffer more with complete anaesthesia. I was hoping not to be aware of this moment, even if to die for a minute but not feel a thing. I'm frightened! I am awake. Their eyes have so much love. Their many years in surgery have not removed them from empathy. Their facial kindness pacifies me. Whatever the epidural did, I start to relax and even start making jokes. The doctor and I talk.

They ask me about my belly dancing and theatre and promise me that I will return to the stage right away because this surgery will be perfect. They make jokes, and I try not to giggle not to ruin their surgery. I hum to pass the time, and get complimented. Lies, I'm not good at signing. But they are kind.

When they remove him, they take him away and say he is a wonderful boy. As my murky mind is carted into the recovery ward, its bright lights knock me into clarity. It's an imposing sensory banging me back to reality. It all happened so fast. Contractions, baby falling out and surgery—the difference between two mothers. Hers was on the floor mine was on a surgery table. A few minutes of warning gave me a different outcome.

As I am carted like a carcass into surgery as time decides to dance around me. It mocks me.

There is no such thing as fast enough. How shall he feel when he finally drops out?

What does death taste like on a dry tongue?

Why are you not running?

Just cut! Cut! No fine incisions to save my son.

Stab that knife and take him out!

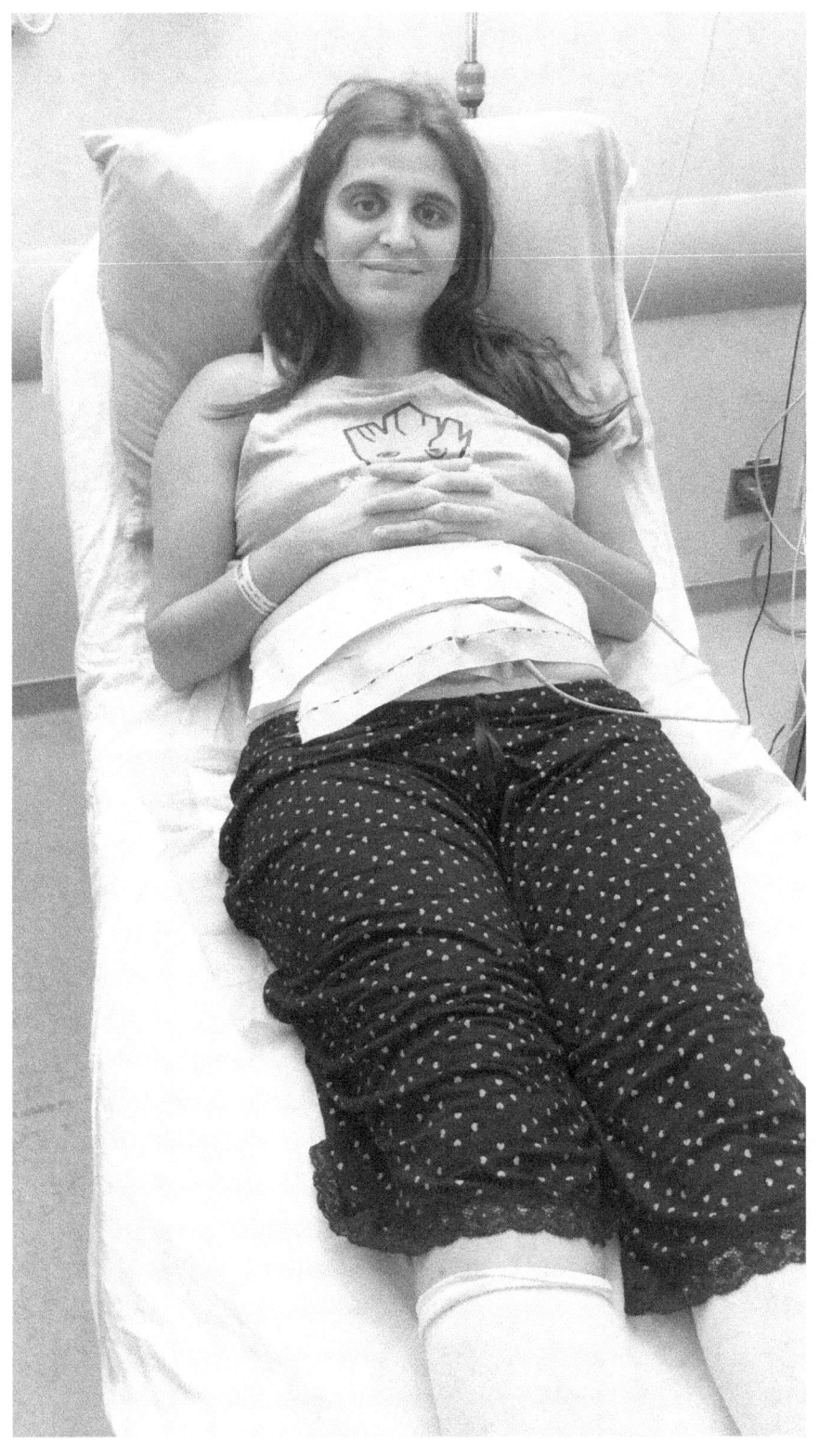

Chapter Two
The NICU

Week 25

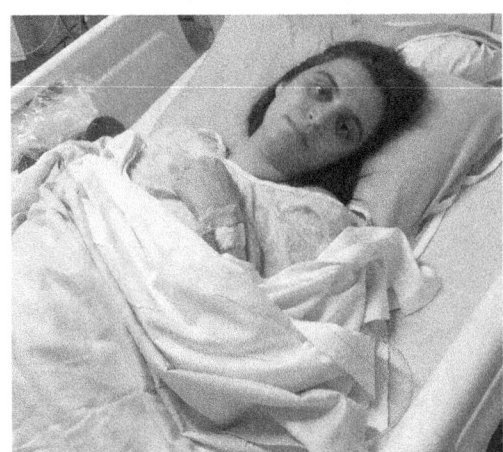 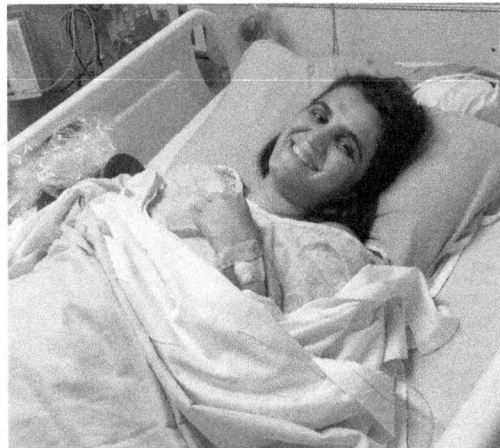

Smile

Sasha takes the camera to capture my maternity moment. She reminds me to smile in case if I want a happy version. They offer her to go and see Elyot while I wait here. I see the fear in her eyes. She looks at me as if she needs permission. We are frightened of what she shall see. What is his shape? His size? How long left as he takes his last laboured breaths? I am in misery to think of him under a bright light somewhere suffering. Now my sister gets to welcome him into an uncertain world as I lie and wait impatiently. I wish Sasha didn't have to see him like this alone. I watch her give me one last yearning glance before she disappears behind the curtain.

 Now alone with my thoughts, I try to understand what this overwhelming feeling is. An exterior force is doing something to me, and I have no control over it. Yes, that is it. It is the feeling that someone decided my fate that I did not want—my son's life and future destiny. Nothing else exists anymore besides my worry.

 A son who is now in his own lottery game. A gamble out of his control over which consequences of such an extremely premature birth shall accompany him in life. It could have been different for him. Now it is all ruined. I get my phone back to call Geoff. We just stay on the phone without any words.

What I did not know at this time is that a dying baby is given to you to hold. They put them on your chest with your familiar heartbeat and voice as they leave this world. Us, being separated like this, means that he is surviving in the other room. I wish I knew this tonight. I shall spend my night thinking that any minute they shall come in to tell me that he is gone.

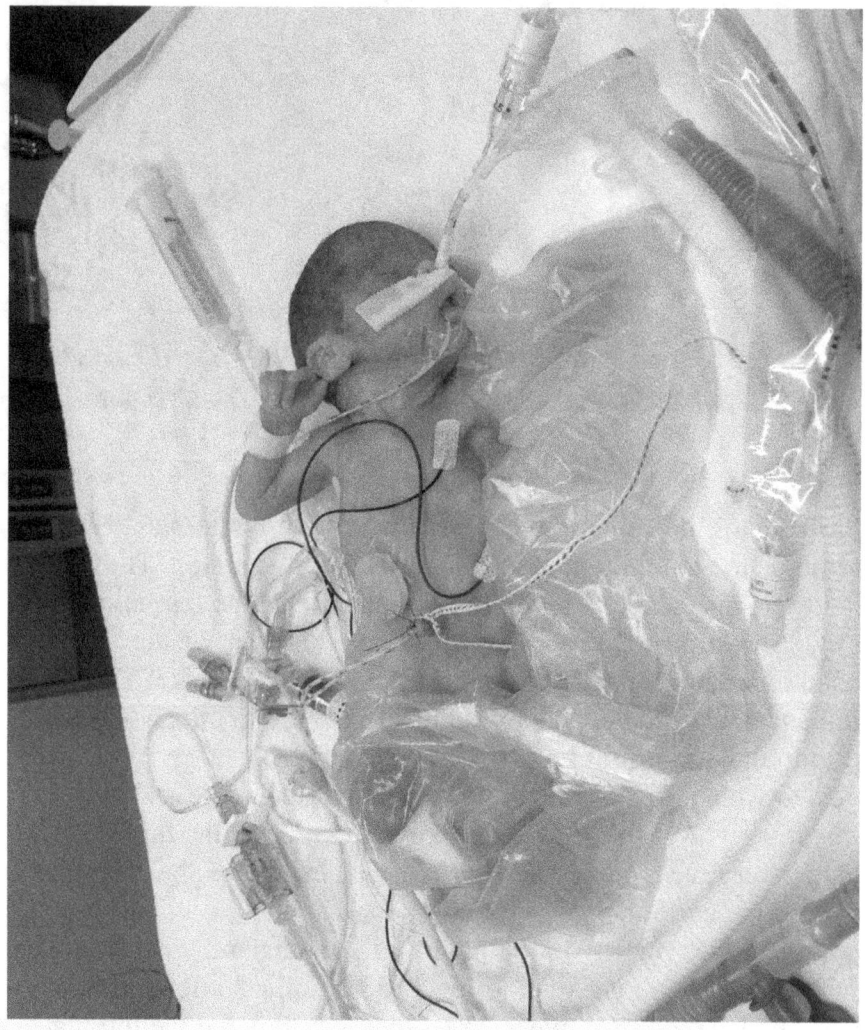

When Maria finally emerges from the surgery room she is making funny faces as she passes us on her mobile bed. Yup that's my sister. I can tell that she thinks that it is funny to goof around in such a dark moment. We share a dark humour. I run right after her anxious to hear what happened.

Sasha's perspective

Sasha's perspective

I approach him as he lies there on the cold table. The nurse motions for me to take a picture. I think that I am looking at the last breaths of a tiny boy. His chest going up and down with vigour. He looks like he survived a burn. I recall this with boundless apologies. The saddest words I ever uttered, "Should I...if he - ". I am so nervous to take a picture because he is suffering so badly. "Maybe Maria should not see him like this and imagine him more happy". I feel so guilty now knowing that I almost did not take his picture. The nurse understands and explains that to a mommy he is beautiful no matter how much pain he might look like he is in. Mommy will love it. She has seen this before. She gently nudges me closer. This is the only time I'd have this moment with him and that any photo would be appreciated forever. She is right. I take a few pictures and videos for Maria. She will want the video. She will loop it over and over again. Always take a photo.

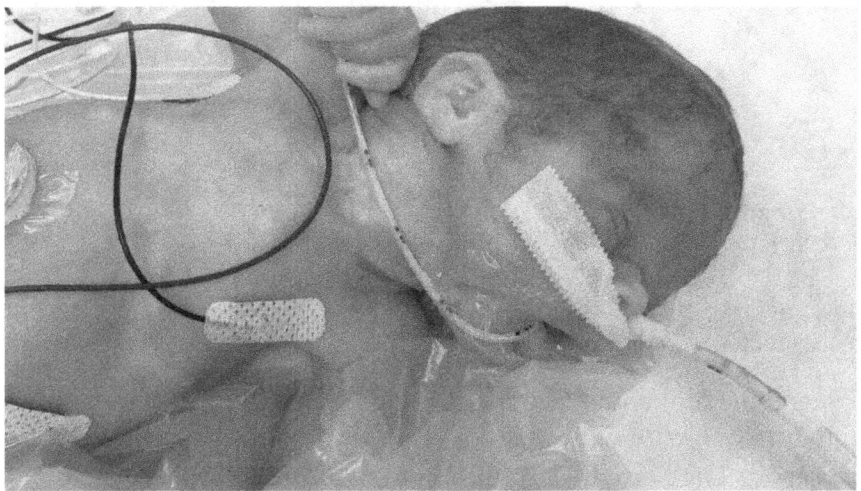

When she returns, she is not as distraught as I expected. She tells me he is big and stable. She sings me jargon of Elyot's strong birth. He cried as he was taken out. A healthy tiny cry that only those surgeons close to him could hear. They got him out in time, and there were no complications. Whatever they told her in that room lifted her spirits. She comes back with a smile and shows me her photos. Her energy begins to relax me a little with the information that neither she nor I understand but is the repeated lyrics of a happy nurse boasting of his birth.

Now they need to watch him for the next 24 hours. I feel a cautious optimism. Cautious optimism is one of the buzz phrases of this place where nothing is promised.

It feels like a walk of shame as they wheel me back on my bed into the Maternity Ward. I feel my roommate's ears on me through the curtains. Their pity is deafeningly loud. It is close to midnight, but no one is asleep. How do I know this? That was me for the last six weeks. They are pretending to sleep while waiting for clues to find out how the delivery went. It is my turn to be a story. It is my turn to make these mothers examine their perils of this ward and realize how lucky they are. They are new patients. All of them missed the death of the other baby a few days ago. I am the most extreme case to them, birth at 25 weeks, at the edge of life and death.

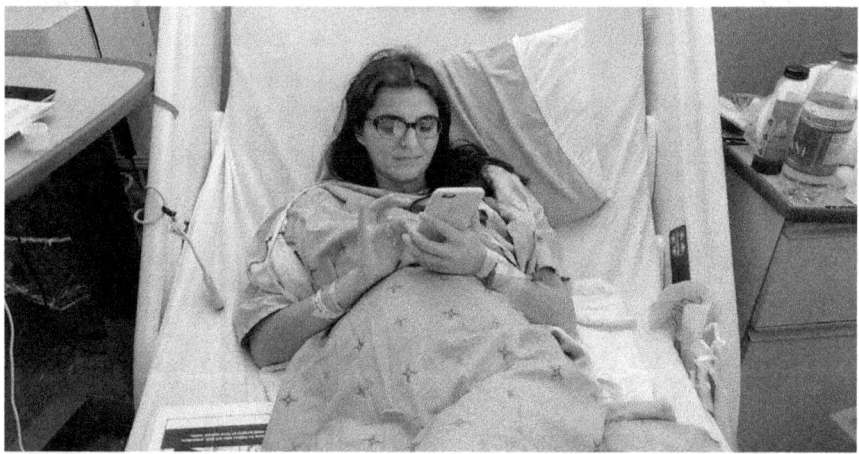

I spend the night studying the short video of Elyot. It shows his tiny torso's breath with the energy of a wet butterfly, quick yet laboured. The body fills up like a balloon through the oxygen tube. He is of a dark crimson tone. I cannot make out the face and confuse the thin eye brown lines for big closed eye lids. It makes his face unusual—a bit non-human. I think of infections. Those can be deadly. He looks cold. Is he cold?

Does it hurt where they pricked you on your tissue-thin skin? Is the light too harsh ? Is it too loud for your tender ears?

Wide Awake

That night I ask nurses for that pill that helps with sleep. They used to offer it to me, knowing that I had gloomy nights. Now they say they no longer give them. It turns out it is for a very practical reason that I discover at midnight two hours after the delivery and ten minutes after I am brought back to my bed. I do not get a moment to relax and have to start working immediately. The nurse brings me a giant industrial age invention of a breast pump and a schedule. She hands over the pump pieces that cost me fifty dollars and the famous chicken bucket to hold all the small parts. I have heard this talk done by nurses to previous patients. Now I am the audience in this one-person monologue show. She is both strict and loving. She is that sales lady. Her pitch is the life of my baby. He needs this milk. She stresses the urgency not to give up.

Flashback to those patients choosing sleep over pumping. I understand it now. Nurses beg, mothers cry. I understand.

I am now in the past, the present and someone's future as they eavesdrop on my very own sales lady talk. I am that person who now likes chicken in the middle of the night. I will have to explain to everyone in the morning that this isn't for food, that it is for my pumps. Tonight these buckets make sense. I put on my foggy glasses and try to figure out the pump schedule. I have to start working on pumping milk every three hours. Like a judge handing down a sentence, this hits me. Do you mean I am to be woken up every two and a half hours to pump? But how do I sleep and forget that I have a dying baby in the NICU? My body still fully numb from surgery. I cannot move but the bed can be adjusted into a seated position. I start my shift. I did not know that you can still get milk so early in the pregnancy. When this realization hits me, I become excited to do this. I thought I lost the milk with this birth. I am tired and inspired.

Pump. Cry. Sleep. Is he breathing? Pump. Cry. Sleep. Would they tell me if he died? Take a peek across the curtains to see if my pump is too loud. Pump for twenty minutes with no results. Set the alarm for the next attempt. Fail to sleep due to worrying. Pump again.

That night a nurse marches in through the curtains. Time stops. She brings bad news. We stare at each other as she tries to figure out my expression. It feels like lightning is going through me. She came to tell me that Elyot is - is - he is -- she tells me that she forgot to get my signature for the pumps. I ask her if my baby is okay and if she came to bring bad news. She realizes and vigorously apologizes for the mistake. We chuckle. She leaves. I am left shaken. Whatever little peace I had is now gone as I worry that the next time the nurse shall come is not going to be for a signature.

It is drawn

That next morning my breakfast has never tasted better. I love the lukewarm tea. I sip it slowly.

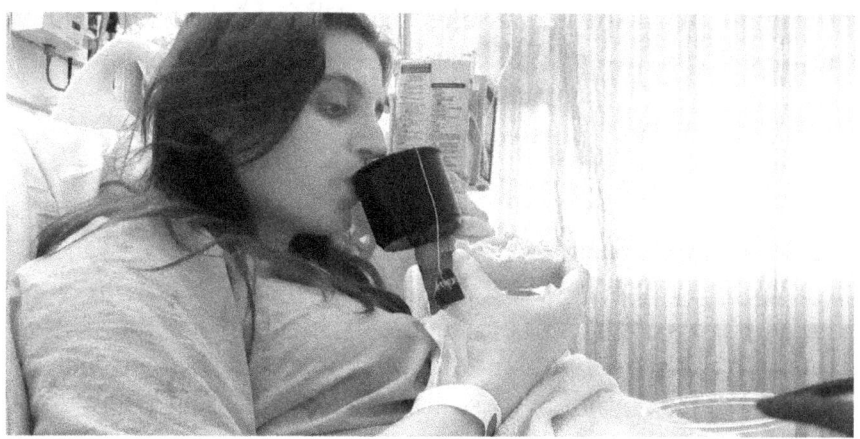

I was in bed reflecting on the night. No one was asleep. Papa told me later how hard mama was crying that night. The whole time Maria was in surgery I was on the phone with Geoff. He was calculating that he might not make the buses and train on time to make it. He was looking at taxi prices that were over two hundred dollars. He was devastated not to make it on time to support Maria and to maybe even get to say good bye to their baby. My husband and I remained on the phone the whole time to keep him company. Now in my own bed wide awake I wished that someone called me. I had to urge to call my parents and even Maria. I had no idea that she was awake and pumping. Everyone was awake that night.

Sasha's perspective

No Celebration

I examine my body. I cannot feel my legs at all. When did they put this robe on me? I have no memory of this.

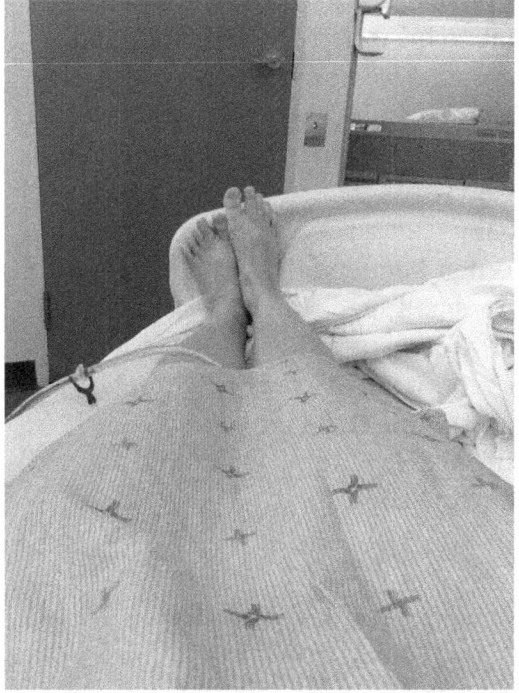

At rounds, there are no congratulations. No one dares to say it. The nurses all understood my anxiety anticipating an early birth. Today they know that I am in despair. Each one who walks in has their awkward attempt to acknowledge what happened while not celebrating it. Some mumble incomprehensibly, others are direct with "so I read your chart, I see there is a baby." Don't fault these nurses. They are wise. At this moment, I crave congratulations, but they do not give it. I am angry at that. I want that talk the other parents had after they gave birth. I want someone to say, "well, this is exciting," as they did with the others. But this is their script to parents like me. They offer no platter of gas-lighting, no silver lining remarks. They follow my cues and play their roles. For some parents who wanted a baby urgently, even at 25 weeks, they might scream with joy. However, for me, each celebratory remark punctures me. These nurses are wise, and I thank them so much for holding their silence and respecting my mourning of what I lost.

***

I begin to shift around in bed as my body is coming back. I shimmy my bum and my knees. I can sit up without support. It was such an out of body experience last night. I recall looking at my legs in surgery but they were not my own. They were numb. I start to remember the surgery now and the details. Will tell Geoff about the legs thing when he comes. He's on the train now. I examine the catheter. It doesn't hurt. When did they put it in? It seems empty. I try to drink more water. Up to this point, no one told me how Elyot is. I am now excited about him. No news is good news. He was a healthy birth last night and is now still alive it seems. I am so excited.

I stare at my pump sheet. It's full of zeros. I guess I don't need my kicks count sheets anymore.

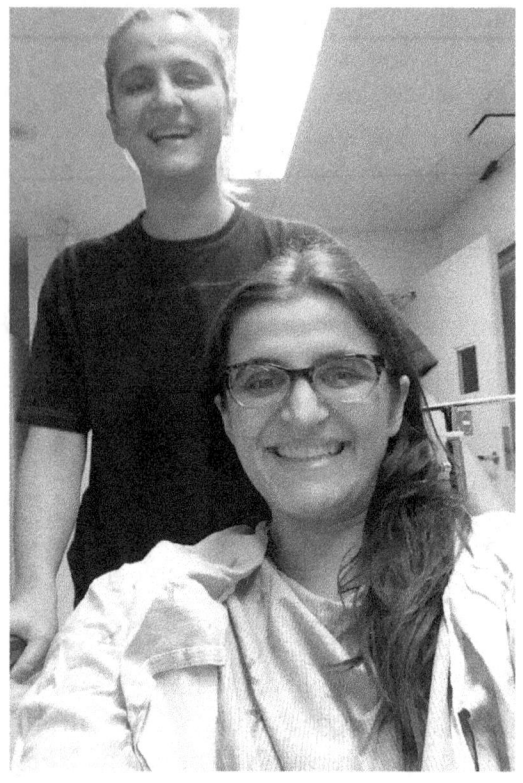

At the NICU I show my ID, sanitize my hands, and look at all their informative posters. They place a 'parent' bracelet on my wrist. I am now a parent. And with an earthquake in my stomach, a nurse finds me and leads me to his isolette. Isolette their name for what we non-medical people usually call an incubator. There he is. He is a bigger size than a 25-week gestation baby; he is the size of a typical 27-week baby – under 2 pounds or 920 kilos. When I entered the hospital, he was on the small spectrum with risks of not growing, but suddenly he is two weeks larger in size. He had no complications overnight. That is good news. He is strong. He is going to survive. I think I have a baby!

It takes us a few tries to get this 'excited' photo to share with my parents. The previous is not convincing enough. Sasha makes it fun. She wheels me around like a race car, almost crashing me into walls. We make a scene laughing, and we do not care. If Sasha is crying, she doesn't show it. She is her goofy, funny self. I cling to the wheelchair hand rails not to fall out, clang! A few accidental crashes do happen.

It sucks that my first moment with Elyot will not be with Geoff but it is already 10 am and he has not arrived yet I need to know how Elyot is.

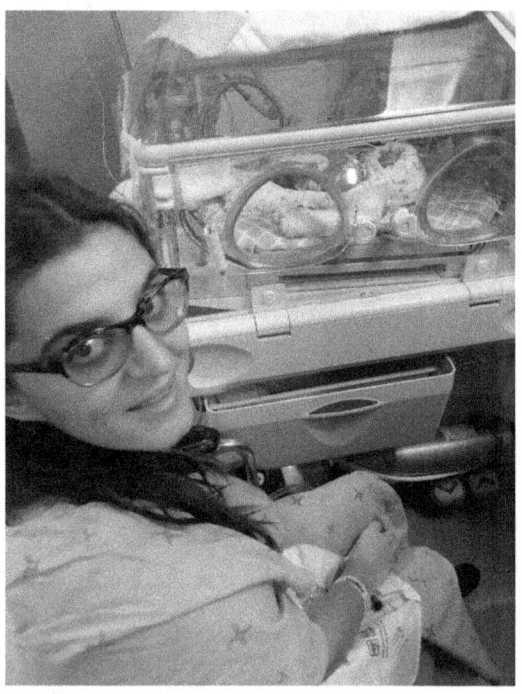

On a side note: Why is my catheter on my lap in this photo? Did I have it out like this the whole time? Oops

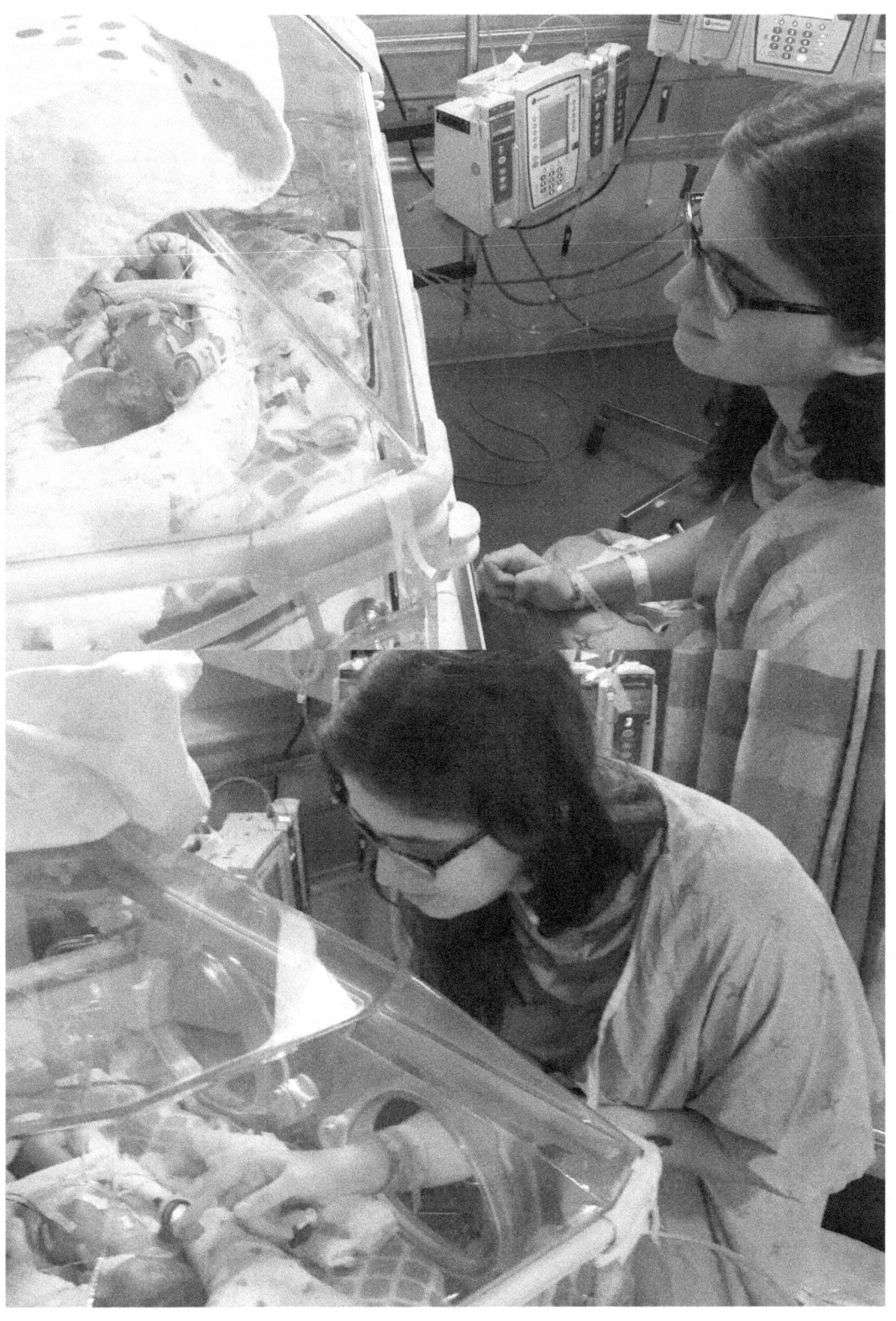

The Touch

What do you feel when your baby is in a glass box? I am feeling faint. I am almost losing consciousness in these photos. It will go away after a few weeks, but my visits do not last longer than fifteen minutes before then. I look inside to see his little face. I want to examine him to explain the mysteries of last night's photos. He is facing the other way. I can't see his face. I wheel around the isolate, trying to figure it out. He is small in a foggy glass case, so I cannot understand what I am seeing. With a squint, I try to make out his features.

He has a giant tube in his nose and a lot of wires everywhere. It looks painful. Does he feel the pain?

Around him are beeping computers with flashing numbers. I jolt every time an alarm goes off. Sometimes it's Elyot's; other times, it is somewhere else. They offer me to touch him. I'm allowed? He won't break? I shake the extra cold sanitizer off my quivering hands, and in I go as if into the mine field.

"Take a picture of mommy." I know the nurse said that because Sasha took a video of the moment. Otherwise, in my reality, the world disappears. It is a loud, aggressive silence. All alarms mute and so do all the people. I am focusing on his little fingers now. His hand opens with a light poke as if in fright, but then ever so slowly settles around my finger. He finds me! Nothing else matters now. I do not recollect this moment. I see it through the videos I have. I see him through this exact camera angles in these photos. Apart from the eloquent display of pixels within this frame, I have no memory. Apparently. I am saying something. I think I am telling him mama is here! I love you.

No memory.

He does not have a name yet. He is labeled 'baby boy.' His fingers are so slow. His every movement is deliberate. I can sense that he is lonely, that he misses me. He craves the sound of my heartbeat. He is confused. His home is gone, and his mama is gone.

Or perhaps it is all me. I miss him. I am lonely without him. I crave his little heartbeat. I spent the last month counting and logging his movements and heartbeats. Now it is beyond a cruel glass barrier, and the only heartbeat I get are chilly numbers on a monitor.

There are two fighting forms in my mind now. One is getting a bit excited that I have a baby. The other is seeing statistics and quality for life. The latter part is more potent. It dehumanizes him. He is not a newborn but a list of challenges in life. No, he is my baby! I shall do everything I can for him! No, he is a list.

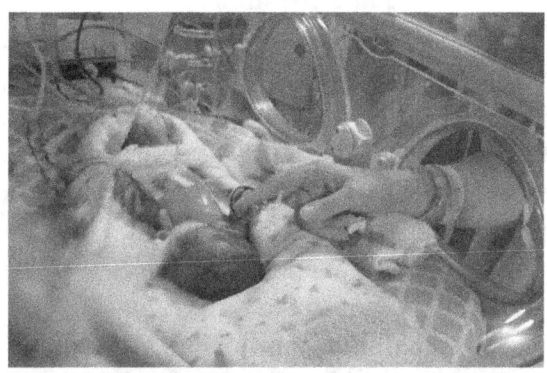

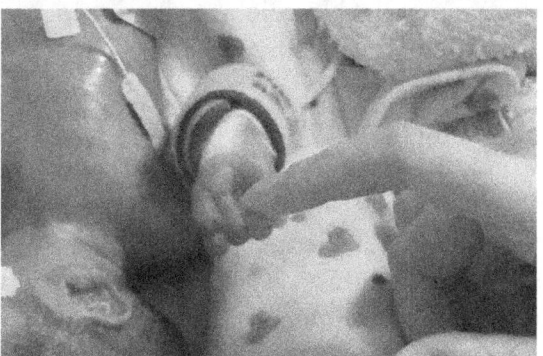

No memory.

How to touch him
He has very sensitive skin, he does not like pokes or pats or rubs. He likes firm holds. He likes tightness that reminds him of the womb. He loves swaddles because his limbs being loose are uncomfortable. He likes your voice. He loves your warm skin and heart beating when he lies on you. He likes your singing. Cuddling him makes his SAT scores better. His heart is more stable and there are less apnea alarms happening with his breathing. They say his deepest sleep happens when sleeping on you. His smell makes me drowsy. He will put to sleep anyone who holds him. His little feet fidget on your tummy under the blanket. He makes me high. I go into a state of euphoria with him so close.

Oxygen therapies:
Ventilator-Breathing tube inserted into Elyot's nostrils that breaths fully on behalf of Elyot.
C PAP – is breathing mask over the nose and is less invasive. Usually for stronger babies.
Nasal Cannula – tiny tube on face, prongs in nostrils. It gives minimal support to babies who can almost breathe on their own.

Papa Moment

Geoff finally drives in from Yorkton, taking two buses and a train. I can tell he is performing the fake positive spirit as well. We have a second actor joining the stage. Please applaud. His daddy moment happens as he gets a 'parent' pass into the NICU. No gendered balloons, no flowers and stuffy animals. No celebratory people are walking in like they own the place. Not for this daddy.

We find Elyot on a C PAP which is wonderful for micro preemies because he is breathing stronger than expected. They like to challenge the babies here and give them less oxygen assistance if the baby can tolerate it. This is terrific news. C PAP is not in the body and reduces chances of deadly infections or random brain bleeds from stress. They tell us he shall eventually return to the ventilator as he gets too tired to breathe.

Geoff's Elyot moment is a scary blue light. They are treating him for his jaundice. His face is fully covered up to keep him away from the bright light. It is like a giant sleeping mask over the eyes. The mask and C PAP entirely hide the tiny face. If I had any glimpse of Elyot, Geoff has none.

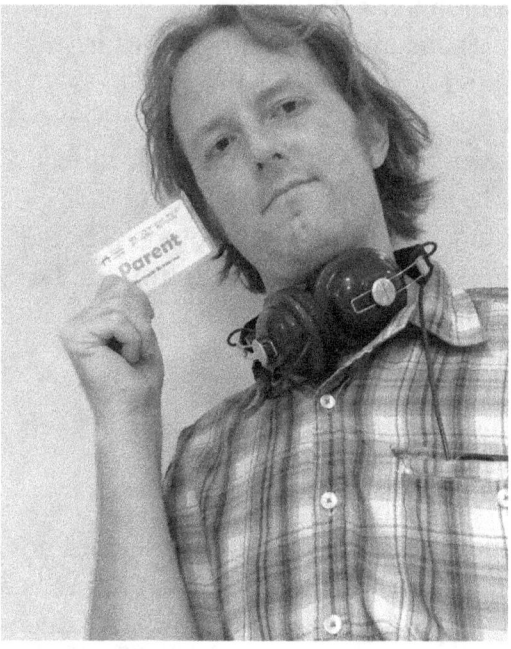

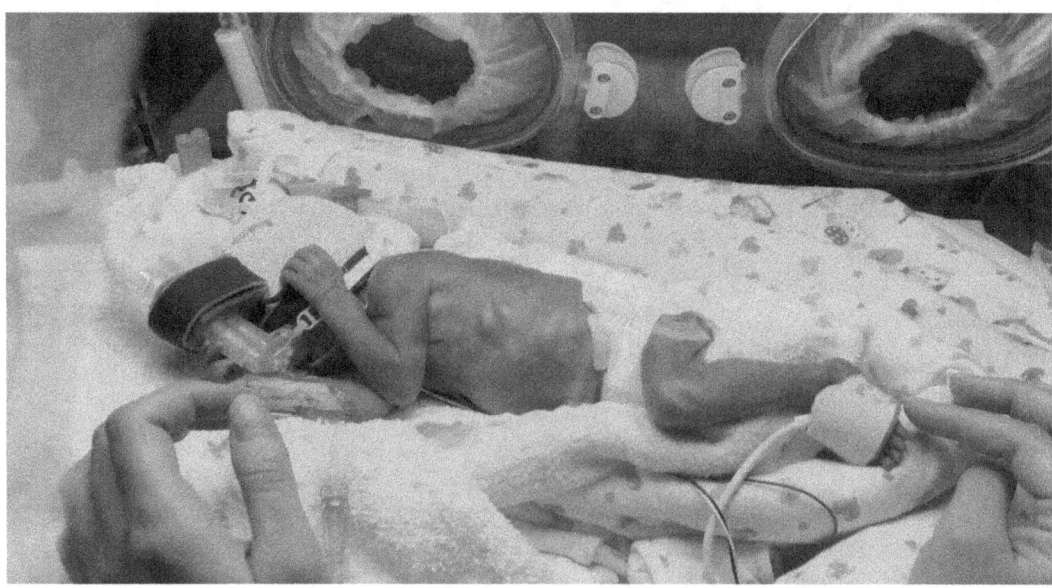

I see it in his eyes, too, those same silent screams. I see his mind channel statistics, charts, those words: quality of life.

In my Maternity Ward time, I only heard them talk of viability, but no one warned us that it would be long term medical repercussions to end us. And even that would be jumping ahead. Tonight let us wait it out to see if he lives.

I think of Geoff's night. I do not think he slept. His train ride to the hospital. How slow is the time when you cannot get here fast enough? I wonder about our conversations. Who would be stronger? The truth is that we both shield each other from pain. As time goes by, I do not tell him about the details of each day when the doctors do their rounds. I summarize that information into digestible bites. I sweeten the grub of truth. In turn, Geoff takes over those hard days when the doctor wants to tell us something. Geoff understands biology and that medical talk makes sense to him. He understands steroids for the lungs and their risk to brain development. He understands the dangers to eye sight the oxygen therapy can have. Then he softens the blow and sometimes even leaves information out. Any extra stress would cause me to lose my breast milk. But today, we are not there yet. Not yet playing concerned spouse roles, just surviving.

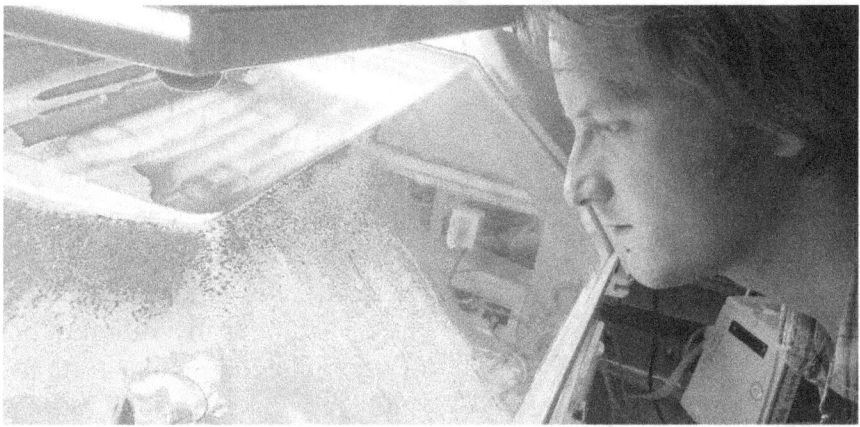

Geoff asks me not to tell Maria yet but he signed a consent form to get breast milk donation in case if Maria's milk does not come in. Geoff is scared that it would offend her and stress her out too early. I watch her struggling with it but she is so happy. I am now worried too that maybe it might not happen for her. So far she is pumping dry.

Sasha's perspective

Pumps

This pump is a premature baby pump. It imitates a sucking sensation like a real baby. It slows down, and falls asleep like a real baby would. Yes, this pump falls asleep! That is a cute detail to which I grow attached. The robot sucking for milk falls asleep. Those first few pumps are dry. They are there to invite the milk. It takes me a few days to see the first drops that I put into the fridge. By the end of the week, I fill up these tiny containers.

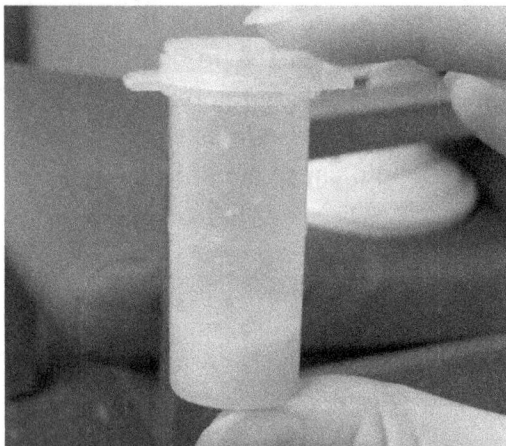

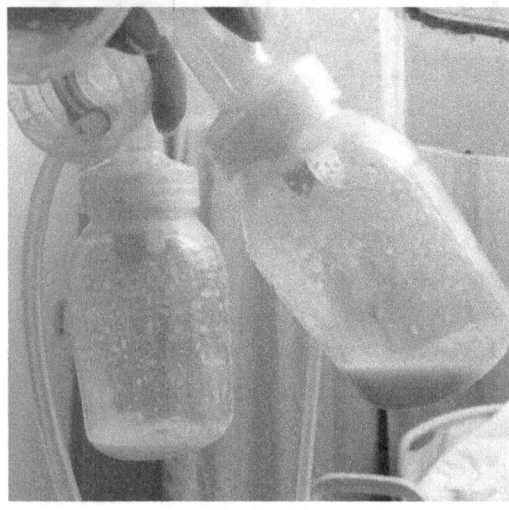

Cleaning them after every pump is tedious. I have barely any energy. During the day, there are Geoff and Sasha to help, but at night I am on my own. I pump in my bed. Then I drag myself with my wheelchair to the sink to clean. I wash them in non-scented soap inside the chicken bucket, rinse, microwave in 60 ml of water, dry with a paper towel, place all the dry contents back in the bucket and go back to sleep. I ask nurses to buy multiples of these pump pieces and keep them in soap water and wash them in the morning together. They say no, there is no such thing as multiple pumps, you only get one pump. There is little compassion for the work parents go through. No empathy. It is what you have to do, so deal with it.

***

The following day we walk into the NICU as he is getting his brain ultrasound. I see his live scan. Large tool caressing his tiny head. One side of the brain is much smaller than the other. The doctor says not to worry because he is still developing. Each new visit, he is in a different position. They rotate him to help with his brain and lung development. Give each side rest. It becomes a fun surprise to see him in a new position with a new cute swaddle. Slowly we pass 48 hours. He is still stable.

Pumps want to sleep too

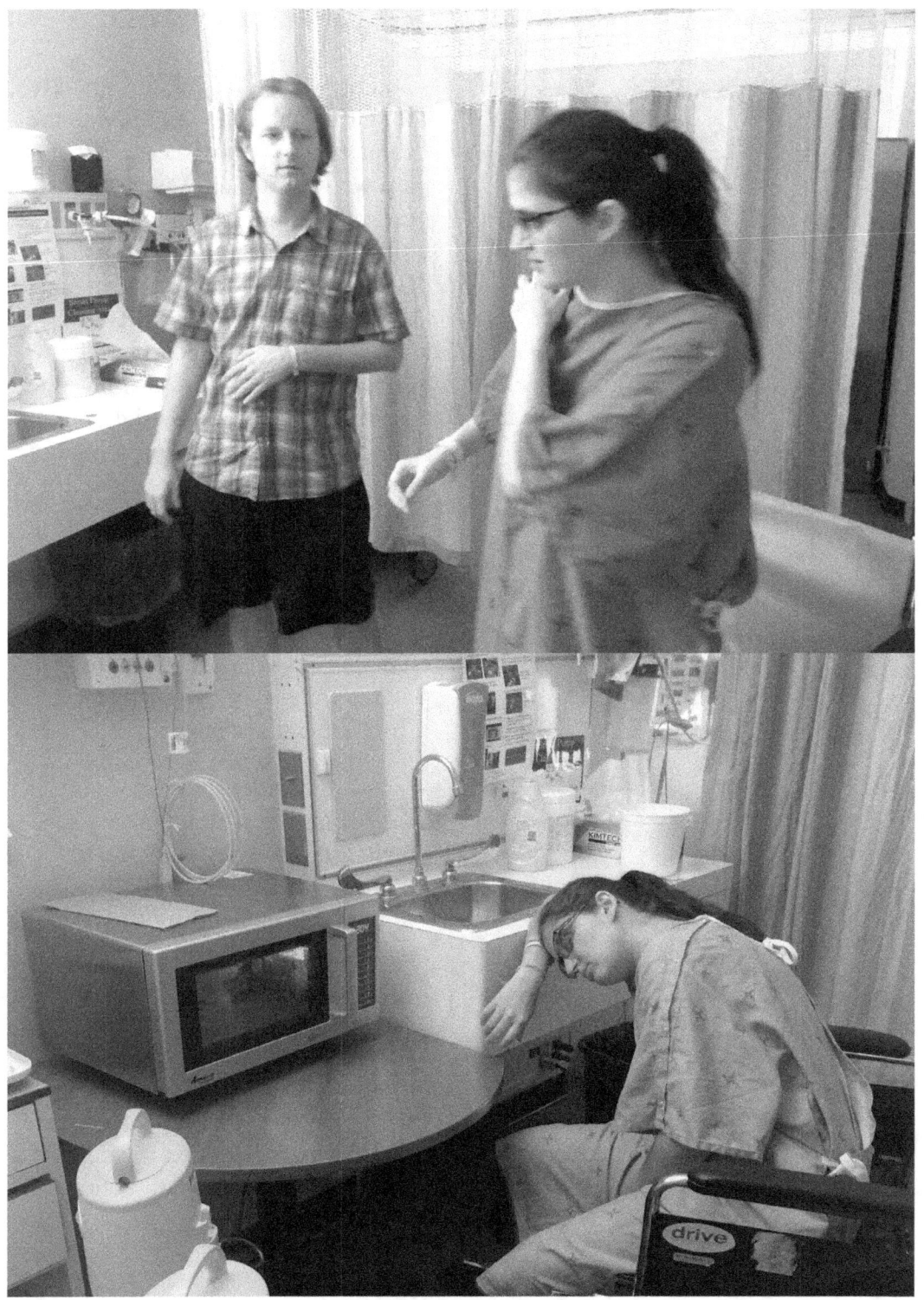

I Find My Wings

Suddenly I realize that if I go out for a ride and get some food in the cafeteria, no one will care. What are we waiting for? I want cake, ice cream, get me everything! If you only knew this joy! I am outside! I find my wings. I spread them and leap towards the cool mists of the skies. No IV attached to me! How I envied those, who were allowed to go on walks. So happy right now.

Why did I not think of going outside my ward before?

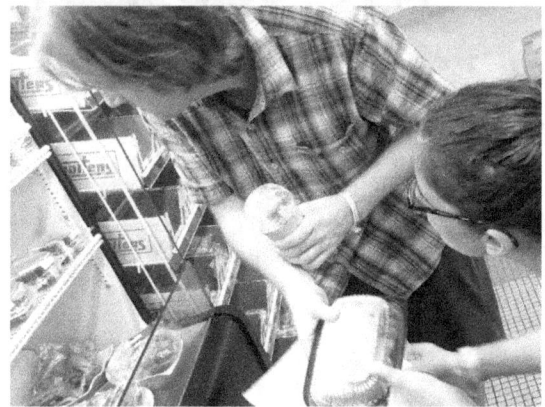

How do you sense the world when your brain is unformed and only in its outer shell. How does breathing feel when there is almost nothing to that lung. When they say it is hoarse and burning red What is it like to be you?

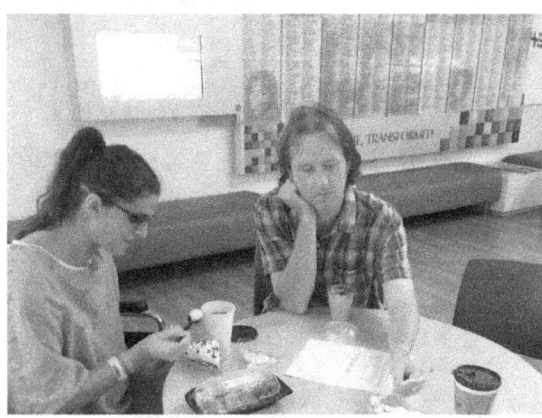

My body is in pain but I try to walk around. They want me to empty my bladder normally and to pass gas. Thankfully I have no complications and it all goes smoothly. In the shower I remove my bandages and realize that my scar is barely visible. I am so relieved. I had a classical cesarean which is reserved for micro preemies and thought that it would be a huge one in a vertical direction.

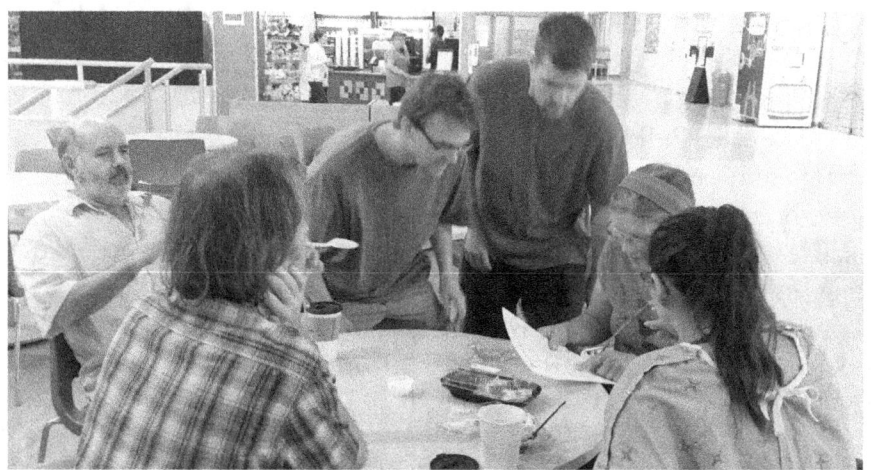

Preparing To Leave

Geoff's family comes in to meet our baby. They help me finalize everything as we get ready to leave.

   I am told that I will have one last meeting with a doctor so I write out all my questions. I separate my questions between an adult doctor for me and a pediatric one. I ask about the expected time line for healing after surgery, what to expect with pumping, which symptoms will make me not allowed to come into the NICU, what to expect at my next check-up. I don't remember all the questions but there were many. With Geoff's family's help I found out where to rent a hospital grade pump. We end up buying a manual pump as well which is an emergency option if my electric one breaks down.

I keep asking all the nurses and professionals the same question. Is there anything I can take for my nerves. No one answers that question. No one seems to have any calming suggestions at all. The attitude is to just deal with it. Is this a gendered issue? That one where medicine ignores the cries and pain of women? You just suck it up. With all the advances that science has made, this issue has been left out. Now I am left with nothing to calm me as I sleeplessly worry about his little life.

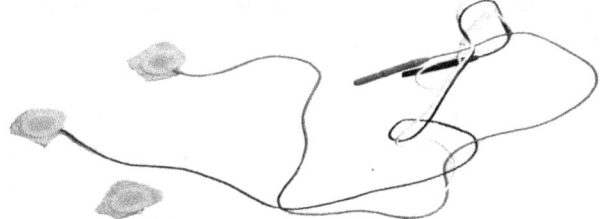

The Viability Talk

Empty dark stage. A lone chair below a spotlight. The talk. Pull up your seat. We all end up here, no avoiding this monologue. It is now Monday, and Geoff is back in Yorkton at work. Only his shaking voice betraying his spirit is present over the speaker phone. I bring with me Sasha for moral support.

Elyot is a micro preemie. The most severe on the premature spectrum. This micro-label shall accompany him through his whole stay here. It shall turn into a curse. It shall become their shortcut word when there is too much to explain. But right now, he is stable though the next 48 hours are crucial. They are happy that he is on the more advanced C PAP.

They explain different things to us and add new worries to our stress bucket.

Respiratory distress syndrome. His lungs are very underdeveloped, are sticky and cannot open by themselves. The doctor raises his hands and cups his fingers into lung shapes, and he explains lung development. It all goes over my head, and I only remember the gestures from this conversation. It is something to do with that they cannot keep the Alveoli open for

> Elyot was born at 25 weeks but his condition resembles a 24 week baby. He shall work through his challenges as such. His history of low fluid adds to his premature severity.

oxygen to enter, so they need medication and synthetic surfactant. The doctor's voice is gentle as he speaks, yet his words are piercing. Later in the upcoming months, they will tell us that he will need different medical therapies for his lungs. His lungs will keep collapsing, and they will change the therapy. They will tell us that the third treatment attempt might have brain development risks. We will worry. Elyot will not need that third attempt after all. Later. Later. It will be our longest, slowest journey. Today we do not discuss these therapies. Today Elyot is on the C PAP until he will not be. Because he is a micro, he shall return to the tube. That label micro is all the doctor needs to say. Because -micro. Not a label but a curse.

Intraventricular hemorrhage (IVH). Words a parent hears as they are subjected to the medical sentencing of their baby. His blood vessels in the brain are very fragile. Any fluctuations in these vessels can rupture and cause bleeding, and that can have brain-damaging consequences.

I attend meetings when Geoff cannot. He is on a conference call but there is often a delay in the message or Geoff is silent. I don't if that's because he didn't hear or if he is not talking because it hurts. I am here for the both of them. During these meetings my role is clear: try remember facts that Maria will definitely will forget. Ask the tough questions. Be the bad cop if needed;. Study Maria's face and preemptively ask for the specialists to cover their comment again; take notes (I didn't take notes)

Sasha's perspective

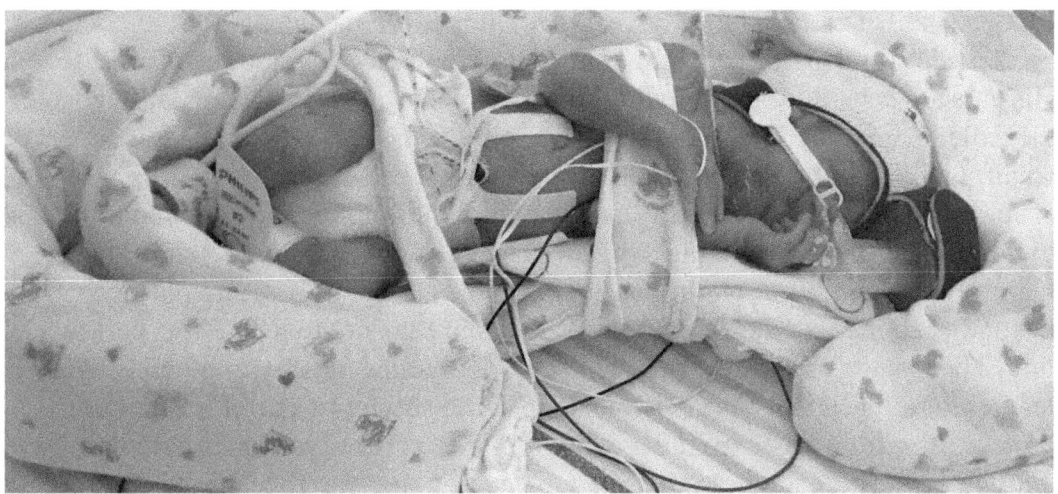

Stress from the endotracheal tube and other invasive procedures increases the risks of brain bleeds and seizures. The endotracheal tube is a fancy way of saying breathing tube.

Meanwhile, they tell us that they are waiting to see if a brain bleed occurred during the birthing process. When they know which grade severity it is, they will counsel us to continue or stop life-saving interventions. I exchange looks with my Sasha and swallow hard in anticipation.

They explain his **PICC line**. It is another thinner tube they put into his peripheral vein that runs through his tiny arm into the body to help with medications and fluids since he is too small for an IV line. It is also an invasive procedure that can cause a baby to stress and get infections and brain bleeds.

Suppose the above risks are not enough. Now we also have the delayed first poop to worry us. Within the first 24 hours, babies have a stool called **Meconium**. It is a first baby poo.

They tell us that if this stool does not happen, he will be in major trouble. Babies have died from this problem. So far, Elyot has not had his bowel movement in these 24 hours, and they are monitoring it. We become obsessed with his stool after this meeting. The blue light. The doctor explains that this very common in newborns and tells us some science jargon to explain why blue light is needed. This blue light looks like a tanning bed. I have never been in one, but I imagine it to look like this. I later understand that jaundice is not severe, but it is my end in these early days. **Jaundice!**

He sleeps. He is not scared. He does not know any of this.

They explain the swaddle. Elyot has a swaddle because these babies like a tight space like a tiny womb. They try to recreate the womb for them. Elyot will struggle to keep his limbs inside the swaddle in the upcoming months. So much for his womb experience.

Elyot's skin is tender, so they have to be very slow and gentle touching him. His ears are sensitive. The windows of the isolette are loud, like the sound of an airplane if you bang them too hard. He can also hear us, so they tell us to talk to him often. It will make him happy. He cannot wear clothes until his body can regulate his temperature. The isolette creates the perfect temperature for him. The isolette also protects him from air-born infections but will be at risk each time we take him out. We are not allowed to be sick when we come into the NICU, or we risk the lives of all the babies, including our own.

The battle shall continue until the very end as each risk of invasive procedures one by one and with it removes the chances of sepsis, a deadly infection.

And scene. Monologue over. Any questions?

As we come to a close to this meeting, they tell us he is on antibiotics and looks good so far. As strange as it might sound, we are optimistic. All procedures have been successful. His heart rate does not show much distress, and his vitals show no infection. We mostly worry about that brain bleed and its consequences on his future but even with that have a strong feeling that he will be fine.

Later I shall hear this conversation with new families who enter the NICU. These nurses are direct and warn of viability. Their facts are cold and sharp like ice on winter lakes. They leave the details for the doctors but make it known to the parents to be ready for it. It is the most intensive part of the NICU – the sick or super premature babies area. Words among nurses flying around here about their tiny patients here are seizures, brain bleeds, cardiologist, and plastic surgeon. I try not to listen. It is painful.

I sit at the table with other mothers in the cafeteria, and I find out their stories. There are babies here with necrotizing enterocolitis where their digestive systems fail and need to be taken out of their bodies for operations. One mother tells me it is hard to return that organ after surgery back into the body until their baby grows bigger. It is attached but remains on the outside of that little body. Their stress lasts months, and I never hear its ending because I leave before them.

Another child who is often sick has patent ductus arteriosus (PDA). That is related to heart problems. I learn a lot about this because a specific doctor has students and teaches them all about it as they circle that isolette. He creates invisible diagrams with his fingers in the air that all the students can see. He tells them about how lung and heart are connected and talks of the blood as something that wants to reach its destination. If I ever go into medicine, make him my teacher. I understand nothing he says, but like his students am hypnotized. That baby will have surgery but way later in his life when he is bigger and stronger. He will have several of them.

Give me your pain

Nothing is Promised

Today they tell us his lungs keep collapsing. I look closely at his chest and see it go up and down, rapid, like a runner. Watching his torso flutter makes me nauseous. He survived his critical 48 hours. Now they want him to do well for a week. Today is the first time I wonder if maybe he might die after all. His breathing does not look easy. It looks dry and painful. I can see the struggle. I try to talk to him, and he puts his hand to his ear. He can hear me! Tears like a waterfall after a rainy season. Faint. Nurses fuss over me.

Taking turns, Geoff and I softly touch him. His vitals on the computer change numbers when we get close. His heart rate goes up when he hears us. Every time we talk, you see it happen. Nurses tell us that he is happy to hear us. I do not understand how they can tell. Later I learn that these numbers on the monitor tell stories. O', these glorious numbers are now romantic ballads!

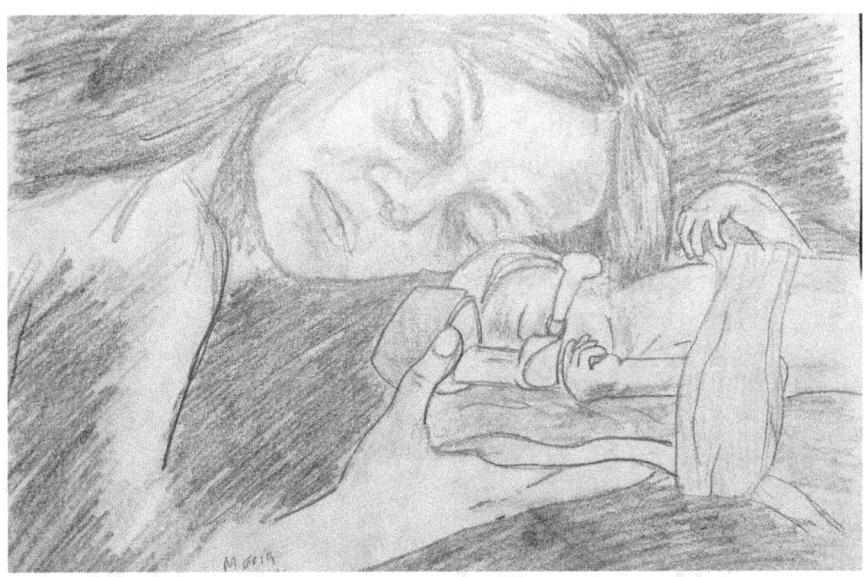

Every time I speak Malerie rolls her eyes. I even give a look of surprise in case she's doing the unconsciously. At some point, she sends her palm out to stop me from talking. She says " yes, we all know exactly where you stand, you can stop talking now". I think that she doesn't like people attending the meetings with Maria.

Sasha's perspective

Home

I smile as I write this. It is such a good page! Thank you page for being here! Today I get to go home. By home, I mean at my sister's house because she lives close to the hospital. Geoff will remain in Yorkton on weekdays because he works there. I am still lonely, but at least I do not go to sleep on my own. I have a house full of family now. We find a place to rent a hospital-grade pump. They do not rent premature baby pumps, only regular pumps. This pump does not fall asleep in the middle of feeding like the previous. I mourn that detail. I miss my preemie pump.

I enjoy having my own room. I can cry all I want, watch my shows in the middle of the night. Also, my milk is now in full supply. It happened to me. There are parents out there who struggle with producing milk. I am fortunate not to have that challenge.

Though the nurses said it is impossible, I do my research and discover where I can buy more pump parts. Actually many stores have these parts. I can soak them overnight and sanitize them in the morning. It would add 20 minutes extra of sleep between pumps. I wish I could find those nurses now and tell them that it is possible and beneficial. I develop a cozy pump schedule.

Geoff and I spend most of our days apart talking through video calls. I do not know which is worse—needing to pump 24/7 and going to the hospital or being far away unable to help and missing Elyot. I think mine is worse, but we do have arguments on who is suffering more.

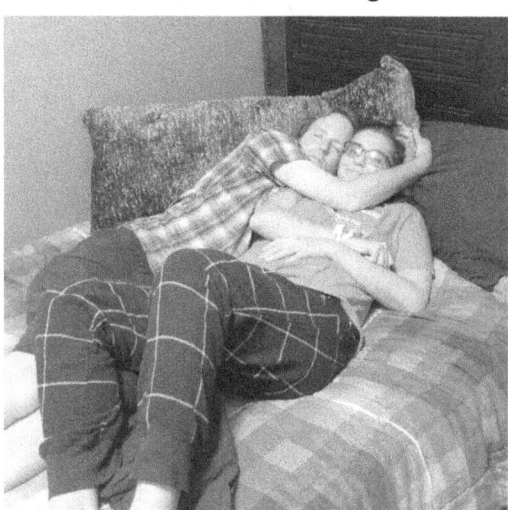

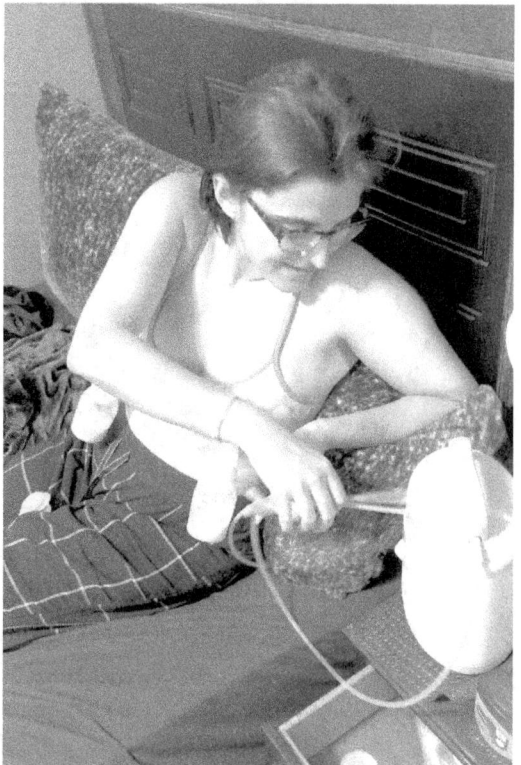

Week 26

His Name

It feels like ages, but it has only been a few days. So much has happened already. If born this week, he would have been a 26-week baby. Still a micro-preemie but slightly fewer risks to the quality of life. I approach this week with anger. Why could he not have lasted a few more days?

We realize that we have not given him a name. Right now, he is still 'baby boy.' There was so much on our minds that we did not notice this before. When we tell the front desk to update his charts, the nurses waste no time making a fun poster to celebrate him and make it feel more like his tiny home. He is almost a week old and still stable. However, there has not been a poop yet. We are far from out of the woods.

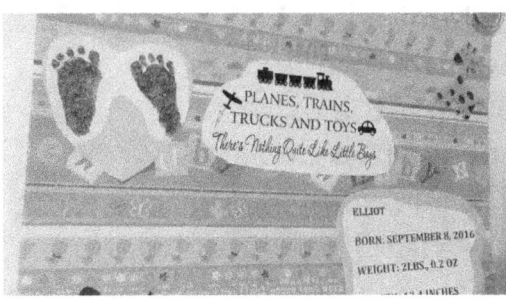

Eyes

This week also he finally opens his eyes. I did not know that I should worry about the eyes. They have to give him eye drops to help him open them because he is delayed in this process. Eye issues and blindness are another risk for babies of 25 weeks. It is called retinopathy of prematurity (ROP). ROP develops when eye vessels do not grow properly. It can happen due to the oxygen therapy premature babies get that causes those vessels to dilate. Babies develop their eyesight in the last three months of pregnancy. Elyot is three and a half months early.

When they start giving eye checks, it will inform them if any changes need to be made to his oxygen. It is always a balance of which therapy we have to prioritize or put on hold. I observe a baby who has this problem but was born at 28 weeks. I watch the doctors in their rounds deciding to slow down oxygen therapy to let the eye vessels rest. That mother is distraught, but I envy her baby being born at 28 weeks. If she just knew my story. I overhear her on the phone with her husband accuse the nurses of trying to kill her baby. People deal with stress differently. But I have seen nurses put their hearts into every baby here. They work impossible hours. Though can you blame a mother when she hears that oxygen needs to be slowed down? They end up leaving us after three weeks. Not sure if to another NICU or the eyes resolved themselves, and they upgrade to Level 2. One day you walk into the ward, and their isolette area is empty.

People disappear.

Back to School

I have to be back at school this Friday to complete my final year. I'm too weak to make it to this eight-hour class only one week after my surgery. I cannot walk to the bus yet, so I get a doctor's note to have this day off. I am hoping that she offers me the weekend off.

> To Whom It May Concern:
> This patient was seen on Friday, September 16, 2016.
>
> This patient was totally disabled on Friday, September 16, 2016.
>
> Additional Notes:
> Maria is not feeling well, she gave birth 7 days ago by C. Section. Thanks for your understanding

However, my teacher does not understand at all. She not only will not give me this day off but suggests that I skip this semester. I was expecting similar compassion as from the previous professor who supported me when I was in the hospital. She deducts marks from my missing Friday, so I force myself to make it to school that Saturday. It is in another faraway city while I am still on morphine and limping in my walk as I bring with me my heavy laptop and hospital grade pump with ice packs to keep my milk cold that I plan to pump in class.

> I am wondering if you should consider taking a short leave from the program to rest, recuperate and provide the extra care that baby Elyot needs. This decision is entirely up to you, of course and if you feel up to it, I support you proceeding.

> Unfortunately, the way the course is set up, in-class assignments can only be done in class with your group and there is no way to make these up. Individually, they aren't worth much so if you miss a day, it won't be detrimental.

There is no crystal tea cup this time. I have no space in my bag with the pump and all the other stuff. The professor does not change her mind about my mark even after seeing how hard I am working. I am tired and barely paying attention. She wants us to write mini-essays that day. I have no idea what I am doing. The pumping machine makes a loud noise, and I feel self-conscious when I turn it on—Bvv bvv bvv bvv bvv. Then after I complete the pumping, I put aside my notebook and start to pour the milk into transportable containers. I label them with time, date and name and sneak them into the shared fridge at the school. There is a shame that comes with such a public showing of my pump routine. It is not so sweet as a nursing parent with a baby but is mechanical and artificial. It feels more exhibitionist to do this. I wear a calm face and pretend that I don't care. If you act like this is not awkward, others shall follow and also feel at ease.

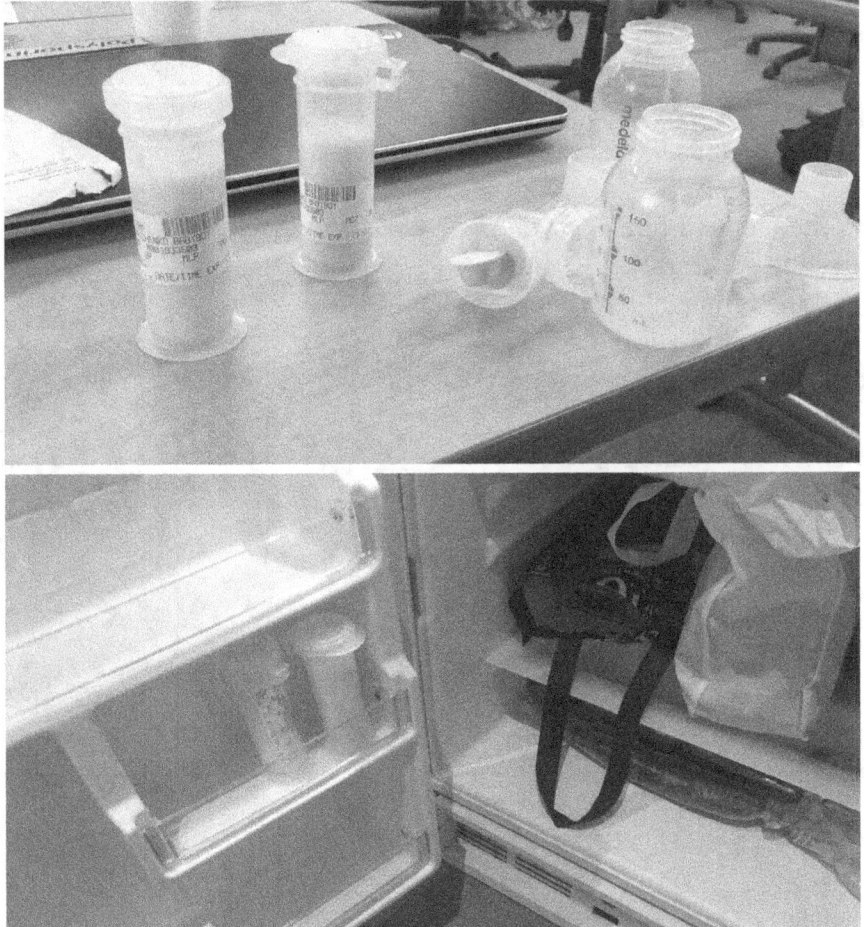

The Cry

After the eight-hour class, I finally return to Hamtown and go straight to see Elyot. It has been the longest I have been away from him. It is now five o'clock that I finally get there. Geoff would have spent time with him before. I watch Elyot's vitals change on the screen as I start to talk to him. He reaches out his hands and starts to cry. Why today? Did he notice that I was not here all day? Or maybe he is just developing and learning new skills. He is so tiny that he sounds like a bird or a small puppy.

I am excited to hear him ask for me and so heartbroken that all the faint is back. I suddenly see how alone he is. I ask the nurses when I can hold him, but he is not strong enough to be taken out today. He keeps crying and reaching out. He puts his hands to his ears when I talk. He is finally present to me. Whether or not he felt like before today, indeed today he has enough strength to show it.

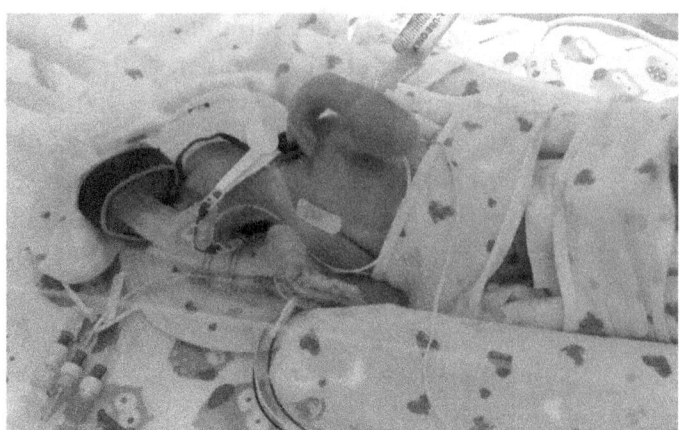
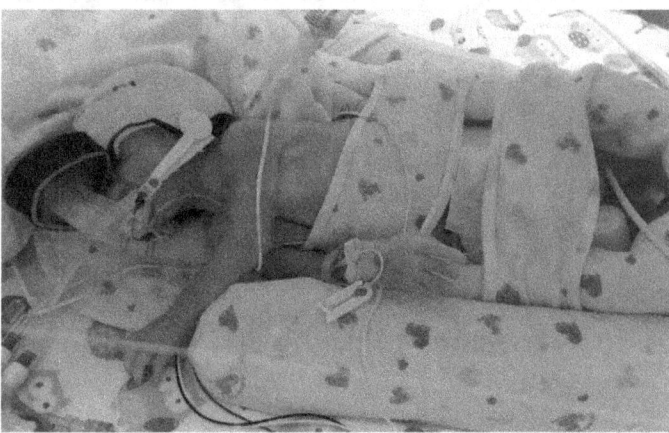
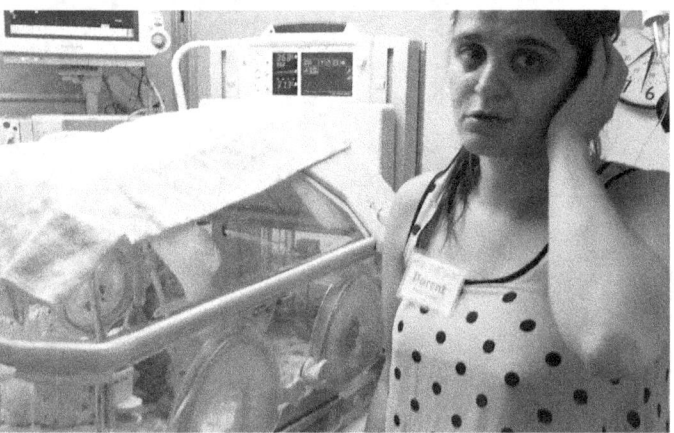

Milestone Photos

Can you believe it is still only two weeks? Each change with Elyot feels like a big occasion. Events up to now have been: being born, getting jaundice, opening eyes, lungs collapsing, brain underdeveloped, no brain bleed, worrying about the first poop (which happens eventually, forgot to tell you), and tolerating breast milk, so they keep increasing the doses. Currently because he is very small he is only drinking a few milliliters worth in each feed. They do not rush increasing it to not traumatize his stomach. Pumping full bottles now there is a lot to save, and to start storing it for the future. Also school is in full swing, and I am already looking into my first assignment. My body is still recovering from surgery, but I am no longer feeling as light-headed at the NICU. Geoff is the same. He is also struggling with sleep and barely surviving at work. We worry about him getting fired if he doesn't keep up. Two weeks. Each event is the size of Mount Everest. I wish I did not have to climb mountains. It is so easy to drown in fear while here: to have burnout. I try to find a way to celebrate all the tiny wins and milestones. I want to feel improvements more physically and not get lost in daily struggles.

We take some of these photos out of order later when I feel safer to celebrate. No brain bleed. We celebrate by bringing in chess. Many babies young like ours will not get this milestone photo but will instead have celebrations more detailed in overcoming their brain bleeds.

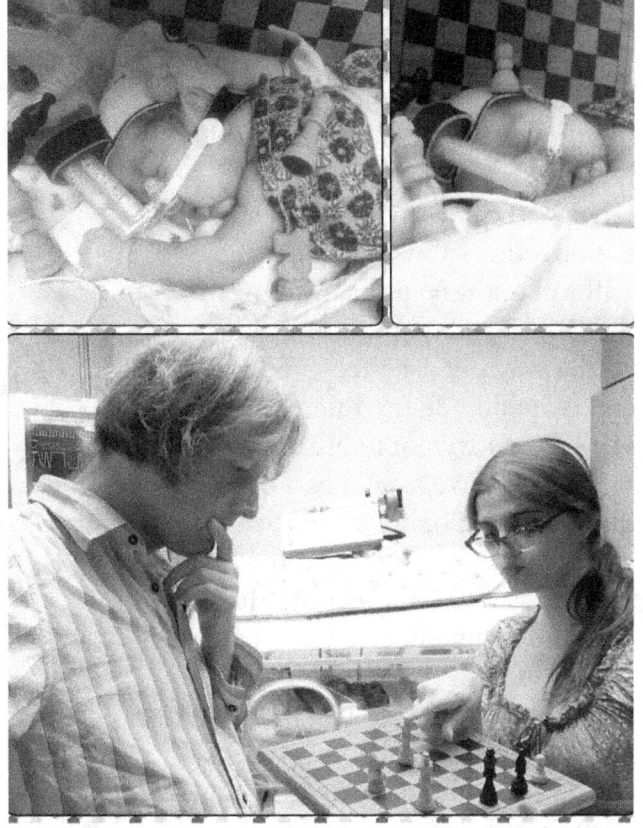

First milestone photo

First Skin To Skin Cuddle

Today he is nine days old. Out of nowhere, the nurse asks if I want to hold him. He is strong enough to be picked up. Yesterday he cried for me, now, he is stable so that he can be moved. It is as if he summoned this strength to get closer to me. The nurse's giant hands gently scoop him up along with all the wires and bring him to my chest. He is crying like a screeching chick. His hands are shaking. He is so tiny that there is no weight. He feels like a baby bird. I barely touch him as I place my fingers on his face. I am afraid to hurt him.

Nurses tell me to hold him still in the direction of his prongs or they will fall out if he turns away from the C PAP and might hurt his nose on the way out. The feet are curling and twitching on my tummy. He is very cozy. I try not to breathe on him in case if I have a sickness to give him. On the monitor, the alarms have stopped. He feels so good that his heart is stable. I hum softly. He has a very drowsing effect. I work hard on not falling asleep. This lasts an hour. As healthy as skin-to-skin is for him, he will need time to adjust when placed back into the isolette. Significant movements from mama to isolette are stressful for him. He needs to get stronger before he no longer feels the strain of being moved. I am so happy to be his home again. It is a beautiful way to end week 26.

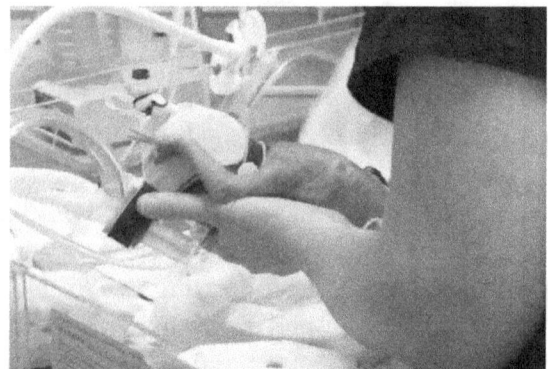
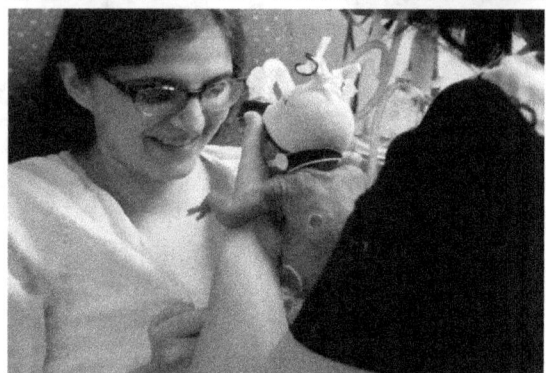
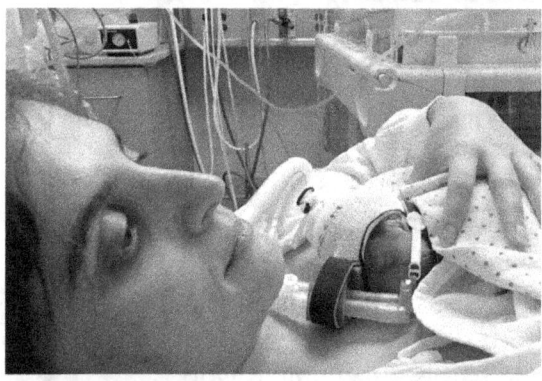
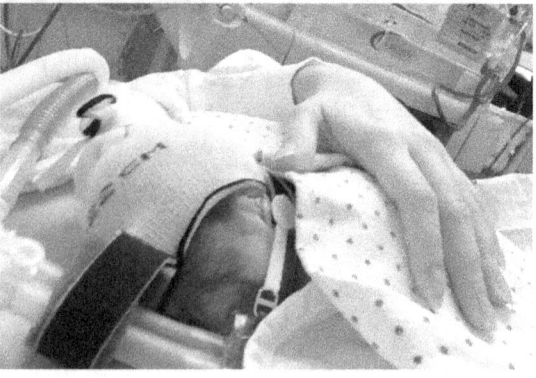

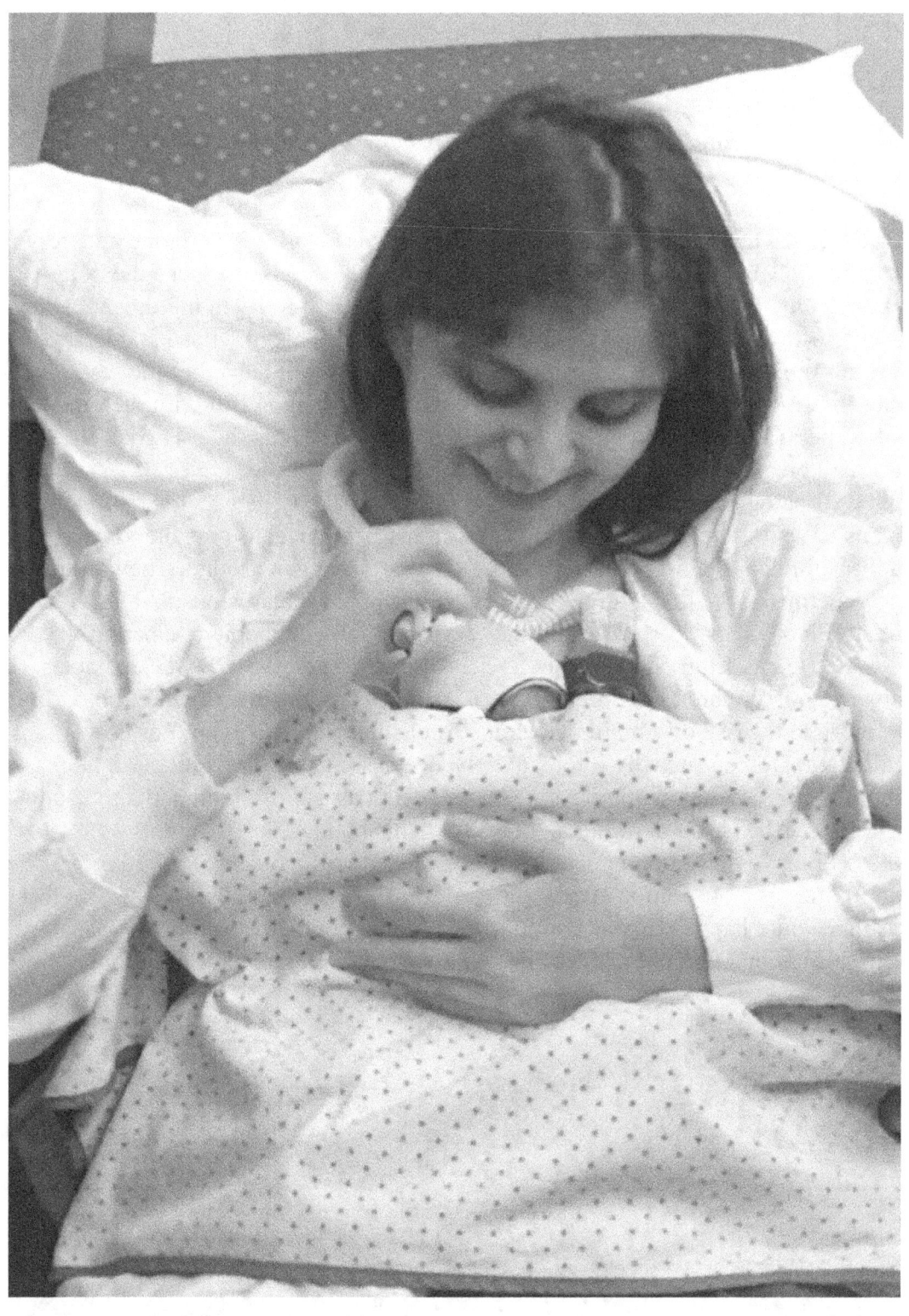

Week 27

Breathing Tube and Blood Transfusion

Trees are no longer lush orange and yellow; they are now getting thin and bare as the weather turns. Week 27 is a strange one. If born today, he would no longer be a micro-preemie, yet it is not yet 28 weeks when most severe life-altering risks go away. It is the transition period. This morning as I rush through breakfast, I call in to ask about his well-being and tell them about my plans to visit. In these early days, I call a lot before coming in, thinking that I need permission. They tell me that today Elyot can no longer sustain the C PAP. He has returned to that invasive, aggressive breathing tube. It is a return to the risk of a brain bleed or infection. Do you see why it took a month to create the brain milestone? These days he is still at high risk of those brain vessels bursting. He is on antibiotics as a precaution. They told us this would happen. It was coming. But this anticipation did not prevent the pain today and disappointment that his lungs are not doing well. I don't cry. I weep.

He is leathery-looking. His skin colour is a dark reddish tone and very wrinkled because he lacks the bodyweight to fill it. Even the tiniest babies bleed. Only his tiny nose and lips resemble a small baby, but the rest does not look human. But with the tube now I can see his face! He has elf ears like mine. I smile.

The next day he gets his first blood transfusion because his blood is unable to carry oxygen around. They tell me after blood transfusions, babies breath better and are happier. Apparently, after a gestation of 28 weeks, babies start to produce their own red blood cells that carry oxygen. For now, Elyot needs someone else's blood to help. Seeing a sack of blood and a red stain on his blanket is terrifying.

Elyot will have three blood transfusions in his hospital stay. This is a low number compared to other babies born so young. Others have a lot more.

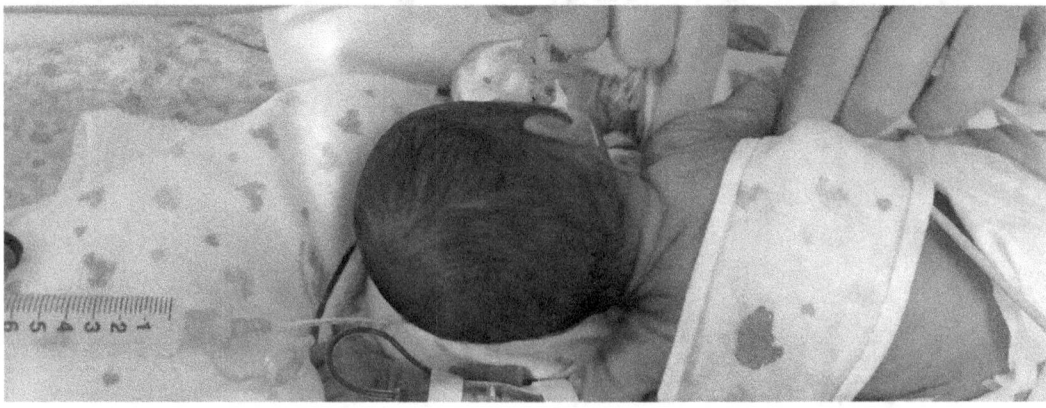

Even the tiniest babies bleed.

The doctor tells Geoff that Elyot's lung treatment is not working. They have to try a new intervention. The third one they hope to stay away from because it might have an impact on his development. He asks me if he should tell Maria? I have no idea. I want to remove the burden from him as well by helping him decide, but I too have no idea what is the best thing to do. We end up only telling Maria a portion of this. She had no idea how bad it got.

Sasha's perspective

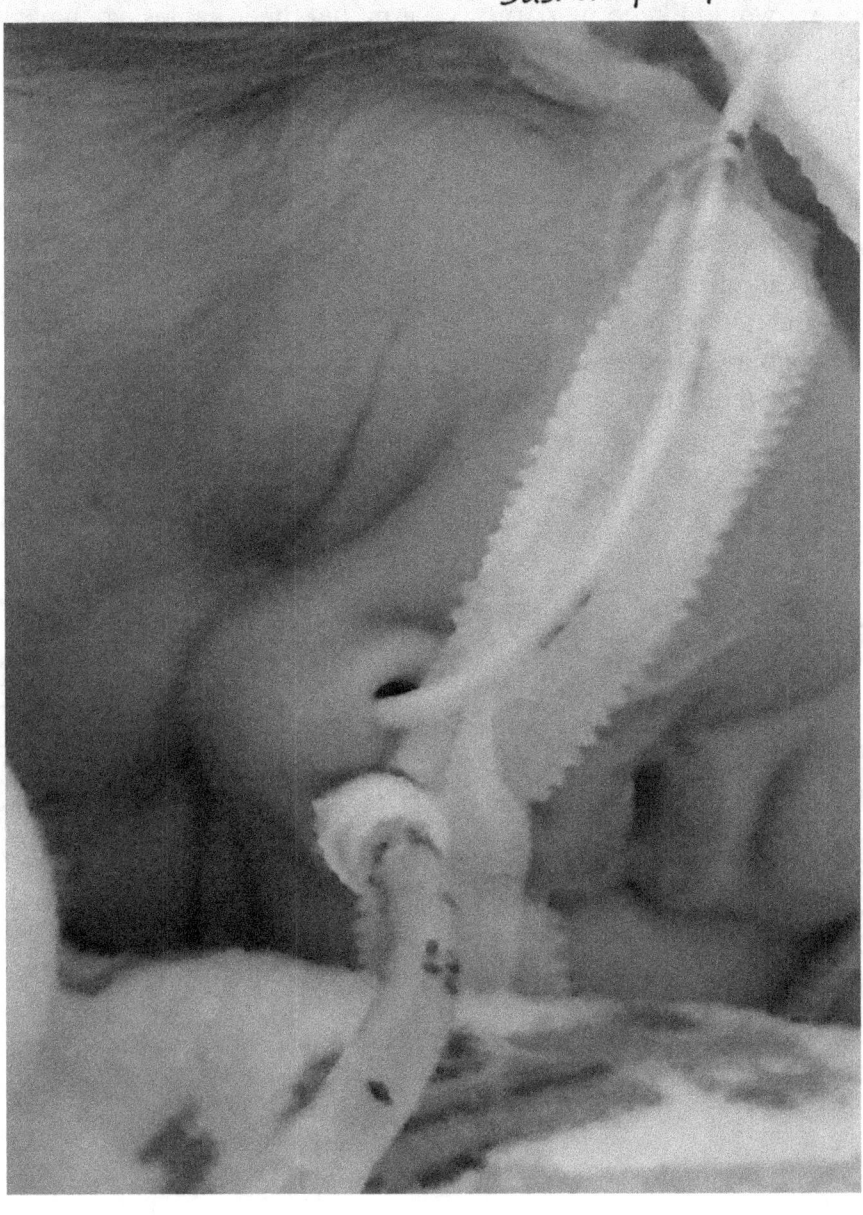

Kilo Club

Today he reached a full kilogram. Nurses are happy with how he tolerates his meals. We take a photo to celebrate.

Newborns tend to weigh 5- 10 lb or 2.5 kg to 4 kg. Elyot, when born, was 920 grams, just under two pounds. Meanwhile, I would like to work on my weight, but pumping breast milk needs calories so I cannot lose weight. I am still recovering from surgery, so cardio is not an option yet. Other mothers walk into the NICU with their big tummies still visible. As much as I want my thinness back, I envy those tummies. I did not get big enough even to get stretch marks. There is not much evidence on my body that I ever was pregnant.

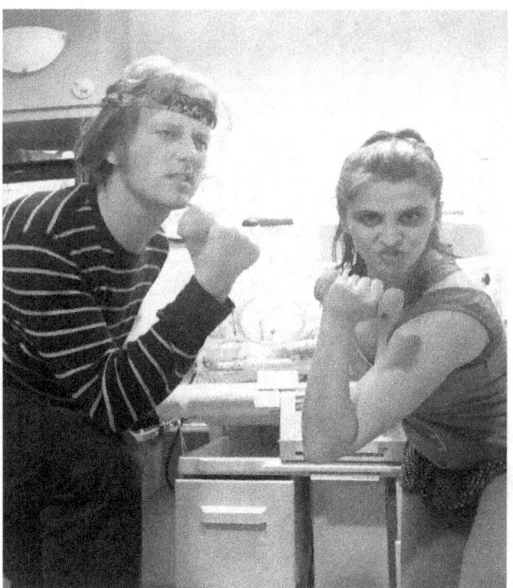

PICC Line Removal

Also, around this time, he gets a real IV line and loses his PICC line. When babies are too small to have veins that can take an IV line to get medicine in, this PICC line tube is inserted into the baby and acts like a vein in the body. Elyot's one went in through his arm, but other babies can have it enter through the scalp and other places. For us, it was not noticeable, but I have seen it on other babies, and it looks scary. It is like a ventilator, while in the body, it poses a risk of infection. Its removal is a massive sigh of relief for us. Photo: These are supposed to be PICC lines tubes on our hair bands.

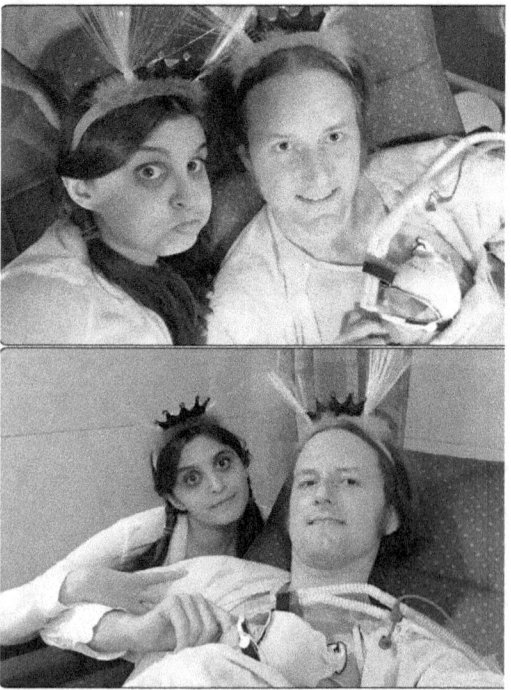

Procedures

Sometimes I walk into the NICU and my walkway is blocked. There are barriers up. It means the baby in that section is going to have a complicated procedure done. I am not a professional and at that time I did not ask about what procedures are done right in the NICU, but the message is that if possible, they try not to remove the baby and work on it right there in its little home.

There are times when I come into the hospital and I see anxious parents pace up and down the halls. Other times I see the team talking to that parent in their special room. They try to make it private but when you have been at the NICU long enough their attempts at privacy don't work well. We parents know everything. .

A couple sits in the parent common area and discuss their baby being at the NICU. They are stressed and trying to find the positives in the situation.
I am tempted to approach them to tell them that I have been here for a while so if they have any questions. I can answer some. I can even mention that I have a micro preemie who seems to be doing well, so will your baby!
"At least our baby isn't a micro preemie. It can be worse! " One dad utters. I feel a stiffness gather up my back and something painful enters me. My strength has been removed that instant. I continue to put away my coat as I was already doing and make my way to Elyot. Now however without any resilience. Be careful what you say on the forth floor. Other parents might be listening.

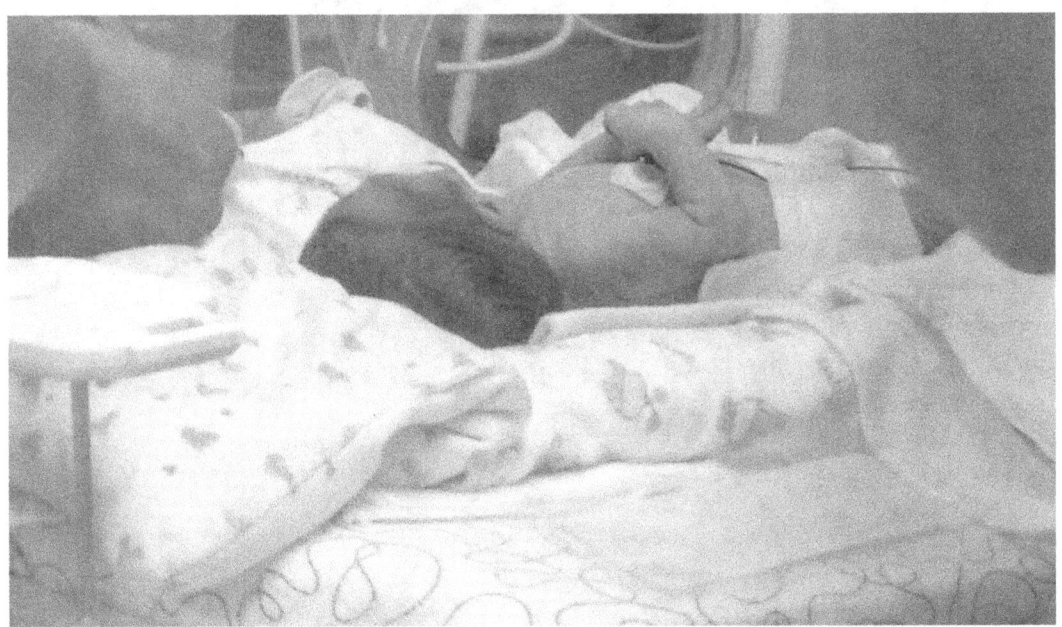

Daddy's First Cuddle

You have to hold him down so that he won't hurt himself with the ventilator. It is thick in a tiny nostril. Elyot is getting stronger, so he is tossing and turning, almost raising himself onto his tummy. The tube limits his movements. One abrupt movement, and his nose bleeds. It is so depressing to watch. I hate the tube so much.

It is Geoff's turn to do his first skin-to-skin cuddle. He is afraid to infect Elyot with a virus. I had to beg him to do a cuddle. In the photo, he is trying not to breathe on Elyot and exhales sideways. A slight exaggeration on his part but this whole NICU experience is extreme. He spends an hour like this with full anxiety while Elyot falls asleep in love. Only the tiny fingers exhibit movement as the body is limp with the happiness of the warmth of a familiar daddy.

Meanwhile, this is the only time I get off. I have many assignments and research to complete for the following week. It is also a time Geoff can ask difficult questions about Elyot's health that I am afraid to approach. He will leave information out, and it is later I learn about how much danger Elyot faced.

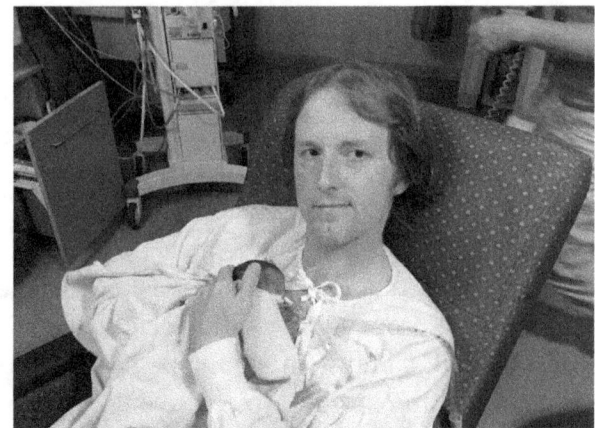

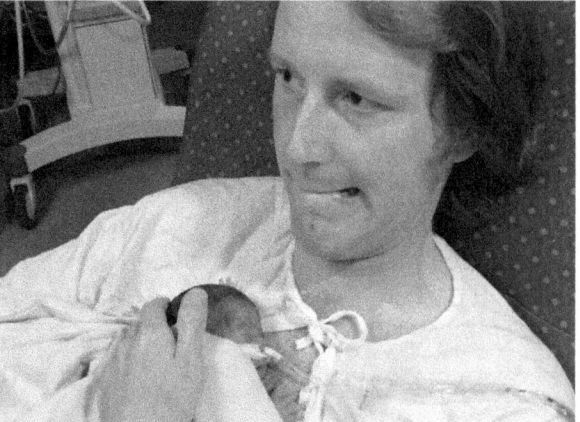

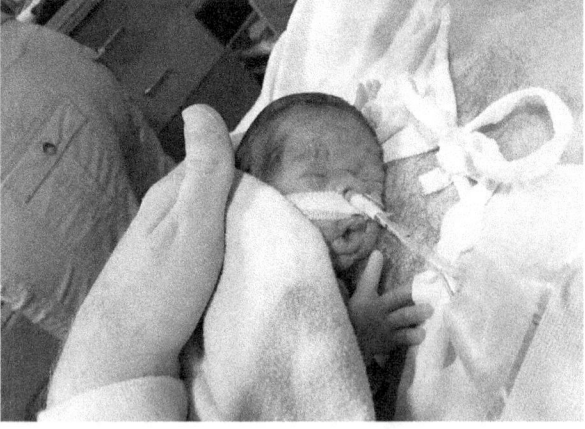

Week 28

Routine

More smiles begin to emerge this week. It is almost a month now. Most major scares have passed. We begin to relax now and settle into a routine. Weeks are still slow, but I notice time pass faster now. Whatever risks Elyot is facing, they are becoming more long-term and cannot resolve within a few days like before. Now is the time to start to wait for results longer. Doctors set appointments in advance as we focus on his future. The calendar is no longer so compressed. Today they are working on teaching him to work on a soother. It is their smallest size. Soothers develop their instincts to learn to feed orally later.

We are singing to him. We did sing before, but now it is more natural and out of joy. He is also beginning to make facial expressions, respond to us talking, and finally turn into a real baby!

Week 28 is when babies are not so much in danger. I thought this would be the same for Elyot but beginning to realize that he has his schedule, not the regular gestation path. He is still stuck within the micro-preemie zone, not at all in week 28 as he would have been in the womb.

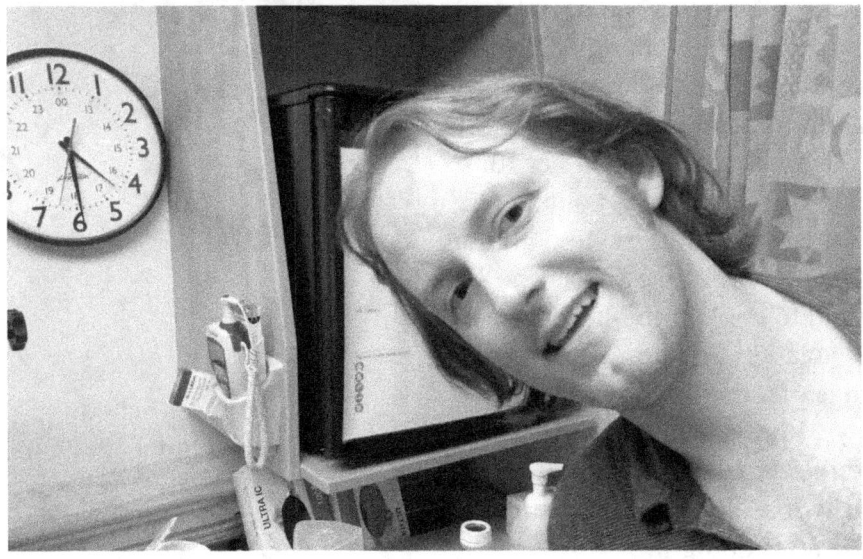

Sometimes when my course is boring, I use pumping as an excuse to leave. My teacher wanted to kick me out for disrupting the class, but I insisted on staying to prove a point. But now I just need to catch up some rest. I find a nice pumping area in a cubicle somewhere. I do two pumps during a given class session. These days are long. I have to travel by train from Hamtown to Yorkton then to Northville. It is a two-hour trip, so I split it up. I leave for Yorkton on a Thursday night, sleep and next day go to school from there. On Saturday, I make that combined journey straight to the hospital with my milk in my cooler bag. So when in class, all I want to do is sleep.

My social worker Malerie refuses to let anyone else come in my place to do skin to skin with Elyot. Sasha pretends to be me and spends Fridays with Elyot. Malerie is a bad social worker, always ruining things. Other social workers let their families replace parents on certain days. Malerie doesn't. The first time I asked her for permission for my sister to come, not only did she say no, but she told all the nurses to look out for the sister who is not allowed to come. I think Malerie sees these classes as an escape for me, that I am neglecting Elyot by leaving on Fridays. I have to pretend that I canceled these classes and that I am visiting Elyot as usual – meanwhile, it is Sasha who is doing it.

Geoff is here on Saturdays in my place. My school has no compassion either, and they threaten to fine me with the tuition for the whole semester if I do not attend. There is no refund. I have to go through red tape to finally get permission to use the university common fridge. Now I no longer have to hide the milks pretending it is my lunch in those bags. It is an impossible lose-lose situation. Assignments are very intensive. I often work on them in the pump room at the NICU, just as I work on pumping in my classes. I am tired.

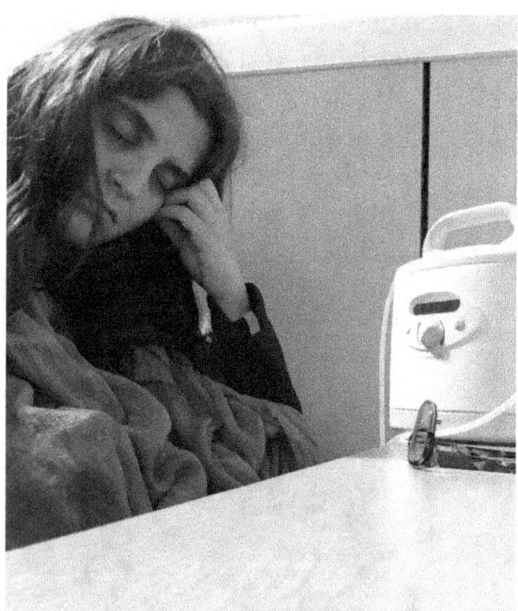

Daily pump schedule:
12 am 3 am 6am 9am
12 pm 3 pm 6pm 9pm …
Every day, every night.

I travel from Sasha's house to my Yorkton home on Thursday night. On Friday I make my way to school. Then on Saturday evening I go straight to the hospital from my class.

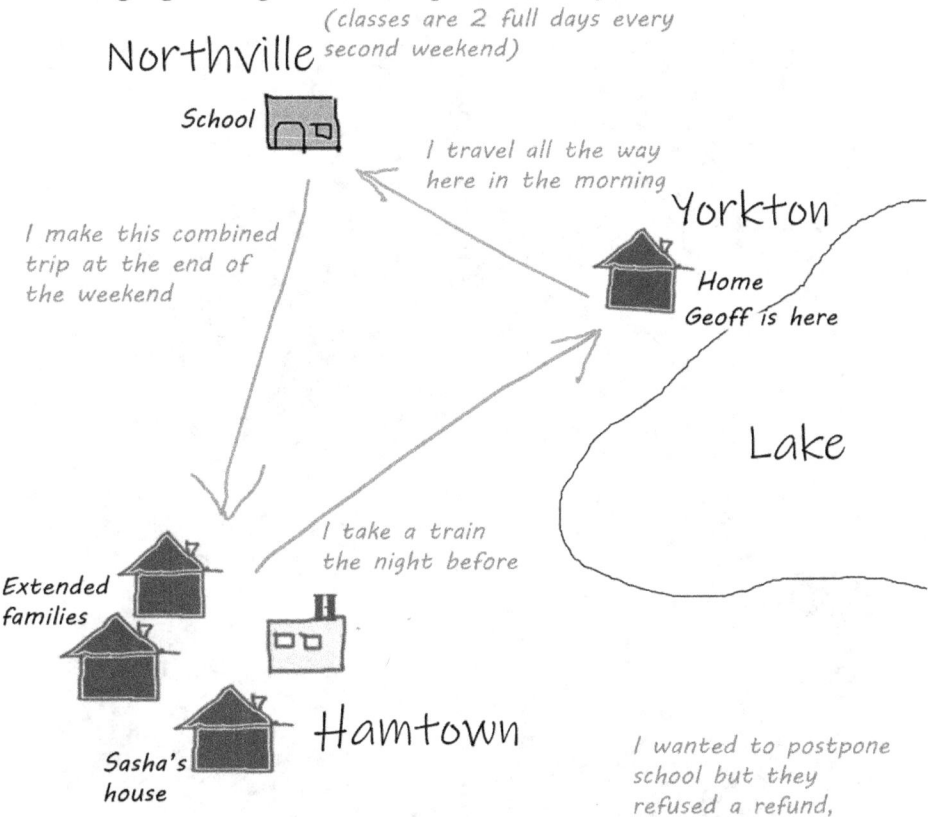

The first week I drive Maria to class because she is struggling to walk. She is pretty much alone with no one offering her lifts. I do my best to reschedule my life to get her to where she needs to be and my husband and mother in law join in to help. Maria is an independent person and it breaks my heart seeing her try to negotiate lifts. She was hoping people offer but they didn't. I see heartbreak in her eyes. She does not complain. I also try to provide her with meals and any kind of moral support but I wish I could have done more. There are times where she has to take buses, I couldn't help. I'm still in pain and regret for those times she had to do it on her own.

Sasha's perspective

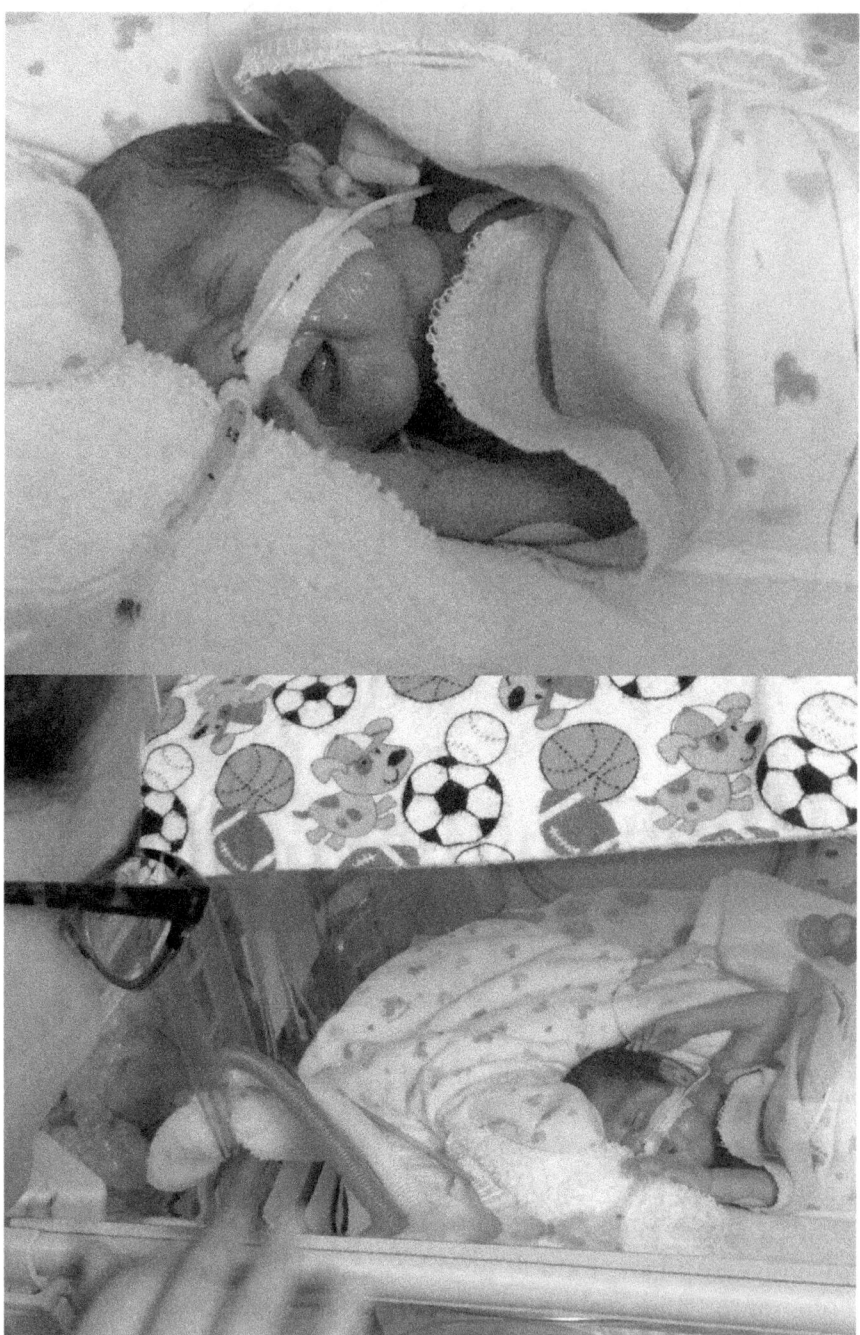

Today you are smiling. You are reaching out your tiny open hands. I sing. I talk louder. If your pain made you far away, now your smile separates us even further.

Chapter Three
The Waiting Game

Week 29

First Newborn Portraits.

Sometimes I am allowed to open up the isolette for a short time. The excuse I use is that I want to do photography. All I have with me is my phone. Today I bring in little gifts given to us for Elyot. Little swaddles and hats. He is a month old but still so small. I begin to enjoy his smallness and consider myself lucky to have such an unusual baby. Not just anyone can have such a tiny toy of a baby. It is special.

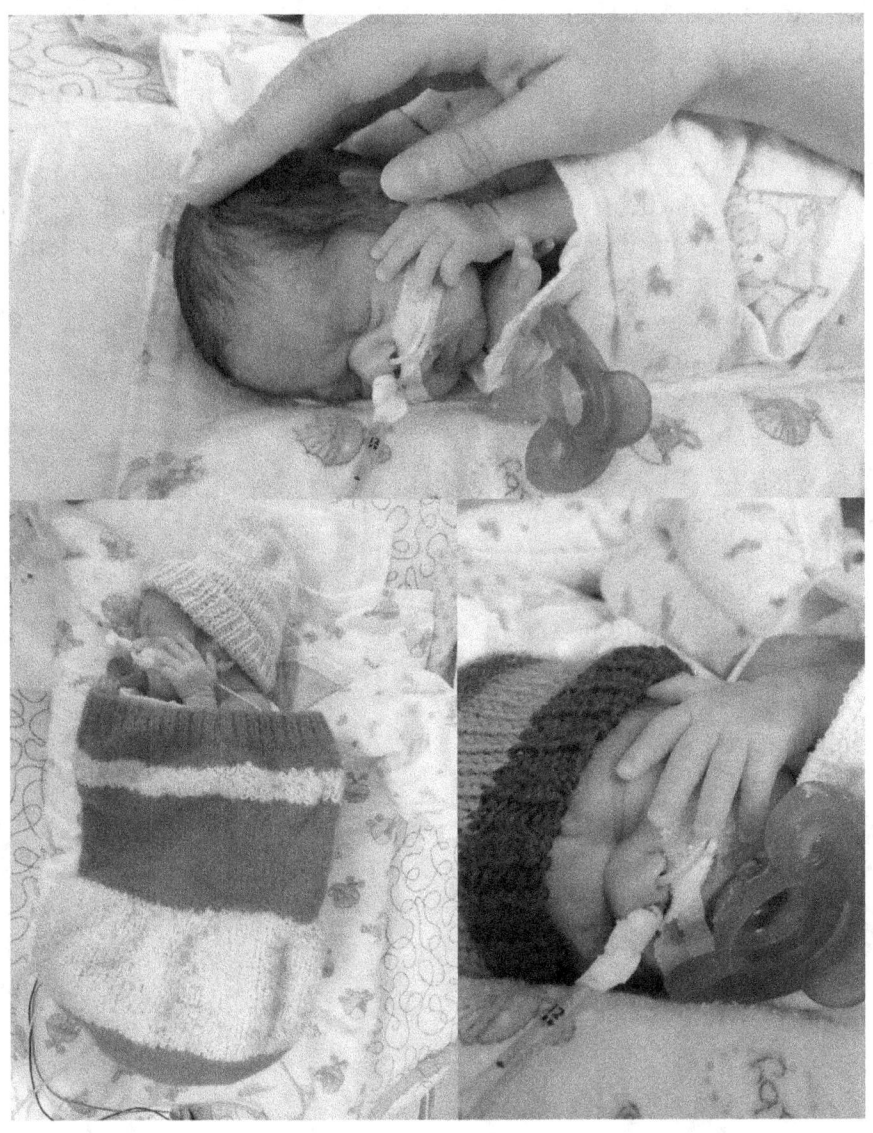

First Parent Moment

I am a tourist. I visit my child in this museum as he lies in his exhibition case. All I do is sit and watch him for hours. By now, I talk to him about everything. I tell him about Plato and the Allegory of the Cave. I tell him about the weather and my childhood memories. I try to read to him, but I am too tired to see the letters on the page. They blur into each other. He is often asleep, but I see his numbers change, so I know that he can hear me. I try to make up for that time when I am at home and missing from his life. I just open my mouth. Regardless of what a day I had, a sleepless night mixed with pumping and assignments. Irrespective of my flu symptoms given to me from pumping. Regardless of burnout and the headaches created from tears. I keep my hand on him, and I talk. Because my sweetness, mama is here.

As he grows stronger, I get to hold him longer. One hour skin to skin turns into almost 3 hours because he can tolerate being moved. I would hold him longer, but he gets handled every three hours. It means that the nurses check on his vitals and diapers then. He hates the cold thermometer that harasses him for a minute under his armpit. He wiggles at the change of his diaper, kicking the nurse away because it hurts his tender skin. He tries to pull his tube and cries because it hurts so much. Handling isn't easy for these babies. They are almost made of butterfly material and have to deal with medical invaders so often through the day. Infections and bacteria can spread very fast in these tiny bodies, so their vital checks are essential to do often to catch any nasty symptoms. I have been a witness to this show daily. I'm not fond of this movie at all.

Up to this point I had limited access to Elyot. But today they let me do all the nurses' responsibilities. I get to check vitals, change diapers and feed him. He is healthy enough now and I have been here long enough that they want me to share the work. I get to warm up the milk and place it into his feeder. I get to open the isolette and … be with him.

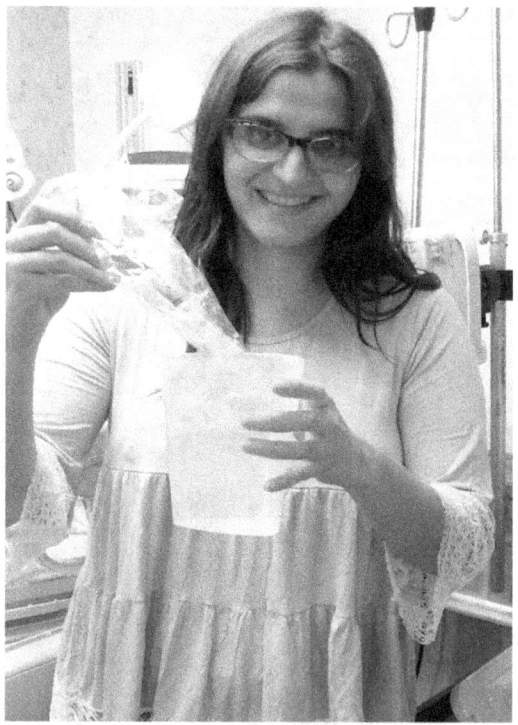

I get to touch him, care for him, to soothe him while he complains about the painful diapers. I get to be a parent for the very first time. We are no longer separated. Today I am with you. Dear reader, if you ever thought you found happiness, I don't know if it can match how I feel today. It is something on a different level. A dream that I did not think I had. It is energy. It is a never-ending smile that my NICU neighbours notice ; they smile back.

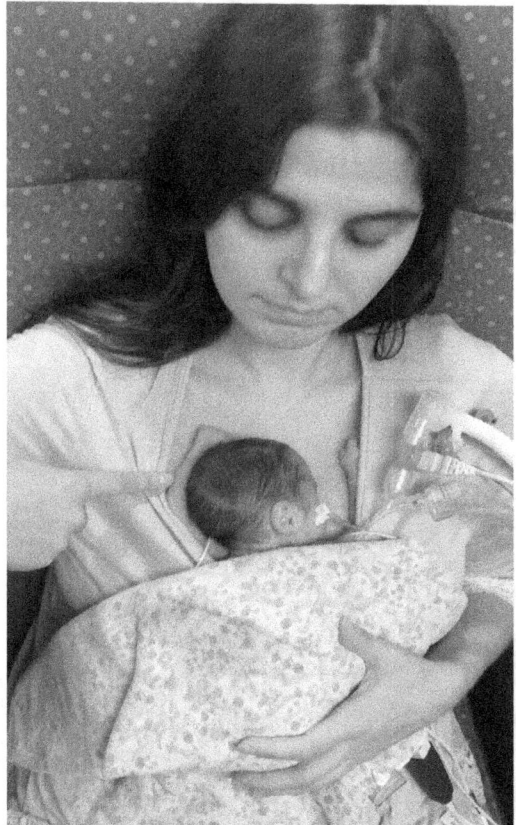

They only allow one skin to skin a day because he gets too tired and needs his energy to learn to breathe.

It is a gentle juggle of keeping old routines while adding more slowly. I am here for an entire workday just sitting next to him, I want to add more cuddles in, but he is not ready.

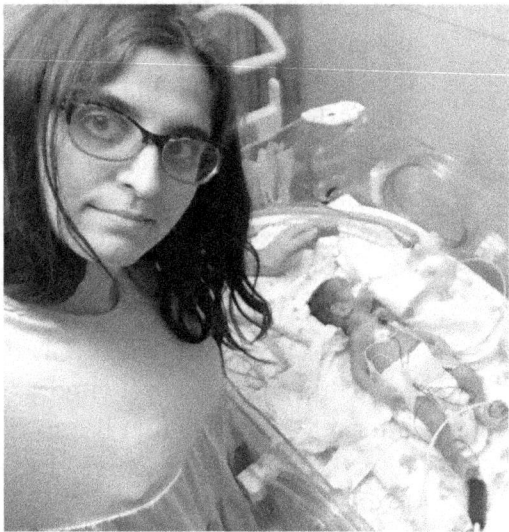

Eventually, the nurses will teach me how to undo his leads (wires stuck to him). Eventually, I shall be able to lift him by myself for a cuddle. Not today, not with this ventilator. But today is the beginning of something new. A visitor turns into a resident.

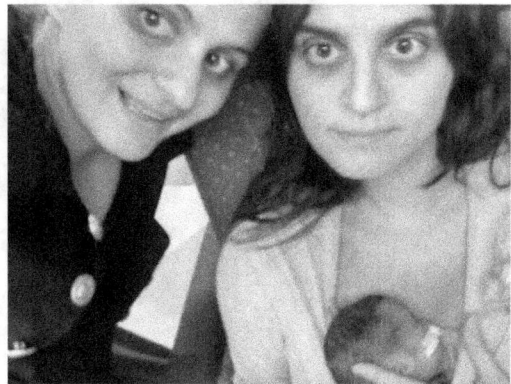

Pump Activism Is Born

NICU is only half the struggle. Pumping is the other half. It feels like organized torture. They tell me that I cannot break this schedule in the first few months, or my milk will start to produce less. I pump at home, in the NICU pump room, on the train on my way to school. I pump even when my nipples bleed and blister up. You deal with it. Attach the pump and let the thing suck you out. At times the harder setting of the pump is too painful to bear.

Engorgement is another problem. If you are late to a pump or did not empty, you develop a rock in your boob. It hurts worse than a bruise. It causes inflammation and flu symptoms. Usually will take me a day to get rid of it, although sometimes a few days. It makes you so cold that nothing can warm you. I try warm baths but those feel cold. The NICU does not let you come in if you have flu symptoms, yet engorgement symptoms feel similar. The internet warns me that if I do not resolve this issue, it can lead to infections and even worse outcomes. Pumping while engorged is the universe hating me. The NICU tells me that most of my milk is being stored because Elyot is only drinking a drop of it. At home, I get special packets and store the milk as well.

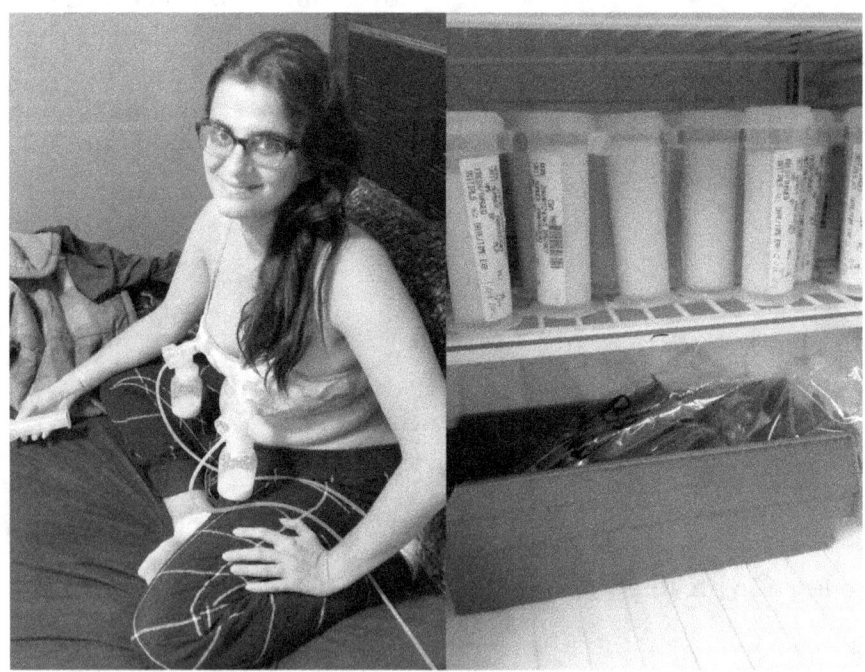

Something happened at school recently. They had a staff meeting at my university, and students from another class made a complaint about another new mother who would nurse her baby in the class. We are not allowed to skip classes, and many teachers will not let us leave to do nursing, so she had to do it in class. Her partner sits outside her class for the eight hours she is there and brings the baby when it needs to eat. Someone complained. Now they added me into this new rule that I am no longer allowed to pump in class. Put yourselves into my mindset. It is over a month now, pumping through the most impossible circumstances to give my baby milk. I do not want to pump. I want to feed my baby regular nursing way. Why do people treat me like everything I do is a fun privilege?

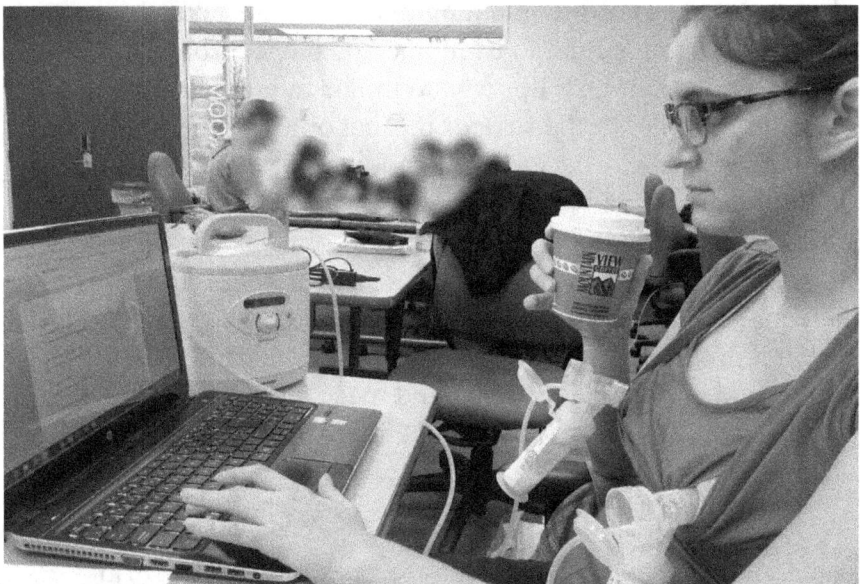

My social worker, at this point, hates me, and I do not know why. She questions everything that I do. She will not help me get a special note to help me submit my essays a day late because she thinks my education is selfish. I lose time when Elyot has procedures, and I spend longer days at the hospital. Sometimes I am behind because of the engorgement flu. I fight for every assignment and do not miss a deadline because we know now that my teacher has no compassion on her end. She, too, thinks I am strange for coming into class.

Now the university is setting rules for working for my son, who is still trying to survive in hospital. Now I am sitting and trying not to cry when the class representative tells me about that phone call.

I start to remember my teacher always offering me a pump room. She would say it is for my own comfort. I realize she meant for other people's comfort. It has nothing to do with me. My classmates have been amazing, No one has shamed me for pumping in class, and I cannot think of any individual who has a problem with it. They support me and empower me. They ask questions about Elyot only when appropriate and do not force me to share my grief. They talk to me while I am pumping. They eat their lunch while I am pumping. They show me that it is normal.

However, this is now something that cannot be taken back. What that committee did to us mothers is inexcusable. I am an entertainer and can fake it. I can do things in public and pretend to be comfortable for the sake of it. That other mother might not have this privilege. I decide this is not just for myself but for all the future nursers and pumpers; I am going to turn this into an activist project. No one will shame us.

I make a very demonstrative gesture of walking up to every student to ask for permission to pump in class. They giggle, fully knowing that I am sarcastic and give me permission. After that, I never skip my class ever again and make sure the pump is loud and proud. I pour my milk into containers taking up the whole table.

One night I was pumping and maybe because I did not drink much that day I started producing less milk then I was used to. I looked at the bottle that barely had milk in it and out of anger I threw the bottle across the room. Once seeing that tiny bit of milk splatter against the floor I burst out crying into ugly loud tears. Why did I throw my milk? Why? I'm so sorry Elyot. I have never thrown an object across a room before, but these times can really break you. My milk was back by my next pump anyways.

At breaks I walk up and down the corridors so that every classroom sees my boob out as I pump it manually. I am slow and deliberate and make sure to pass every class in attendance so that they see me. I make eye contact with each student.

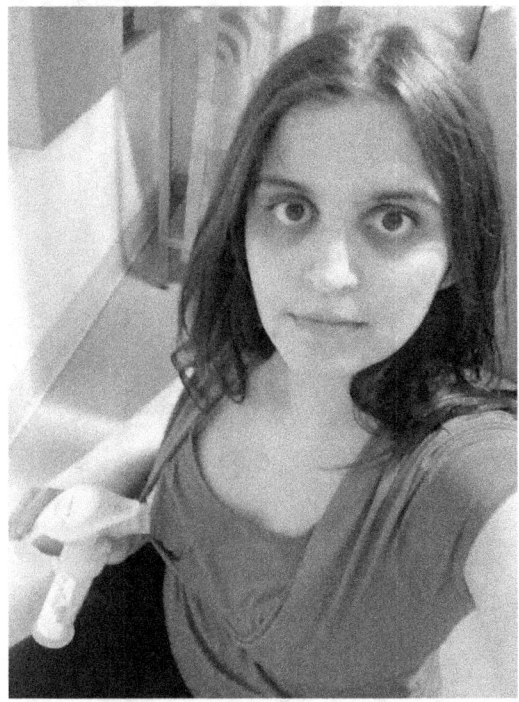

If you want to be offended, I am here to bring it. I am angry now, and to me, you have started a war. I shall confront every human with my pump out to ensure that my eyes eventually meet that villain who did this.

I continue my work as usual, but now I have the energy I have not experienced during this ordeal. I have something to strive for, for petty vengeance against those who complained about us. To start a revolution in this school so that no future parent ever has to be told to leave the room when they are merely keeping their child alive. And if the parent does choose to leave the room so that their mark is safe. It is now a human rights issue and shall become my obsession within these school walls and beyond.

Meet my gaze. I am a proud mama. Look at my pump. It is saving a life. A tiny boy is counting on me, and I am going to do everything for him.

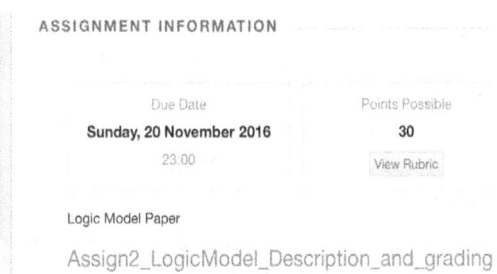

Proofread my work, click the button to submit, pump, submit another article, pour milk into containers, smirk, do a group project with the people sitting around me. Continue the cycle.

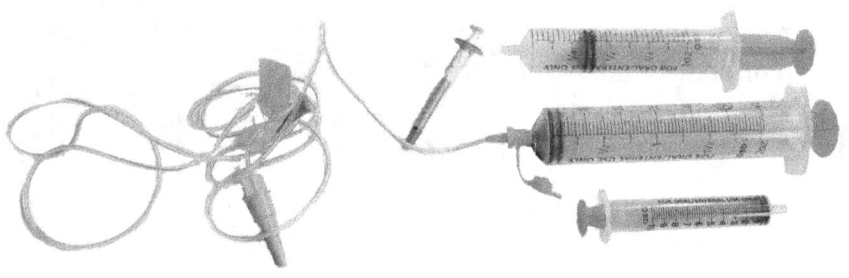

It does not end at school because I start to take this attitude everywhere I go. I pump in coffee shops on my way to the NICU as I grab my breakfast. Secretly armed with clever comebacks, if someone tries to shame me, they don't. I sit eating my breakfast and pump, pretending not to care.

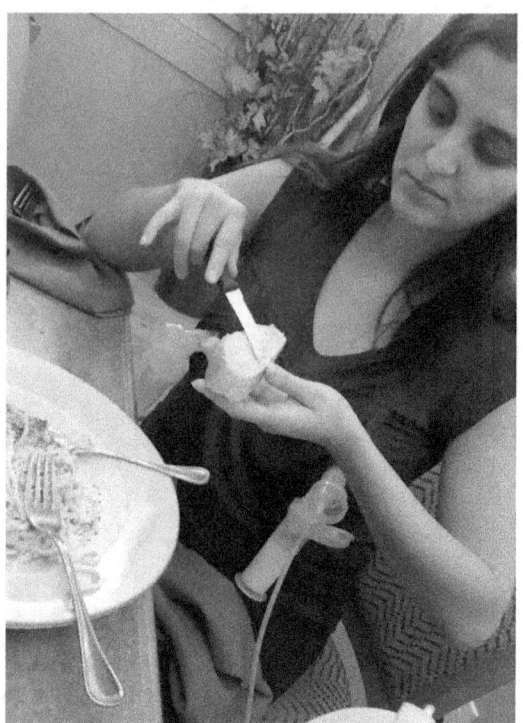

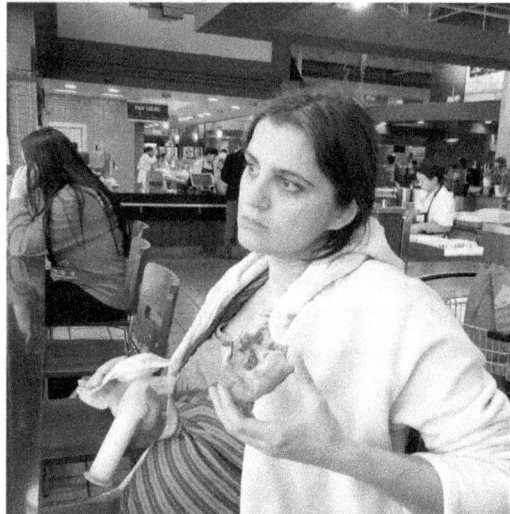

Later I take my experiment to restaurants and pubs. Sometimes it is my hospital grade pump; other times, it is this small manual one. The routine is always the same. I pump and put my milk into their special containers and store them inside my cold pack until I take them home. It helps to have family and friends close by to laugh with me. People either pretend not to notice or are helpful. Waiters offer me water and anything I need. I pump everywhere. I want to offend. Come at me. I want to fight. I'm ready to destroy your prejudice.

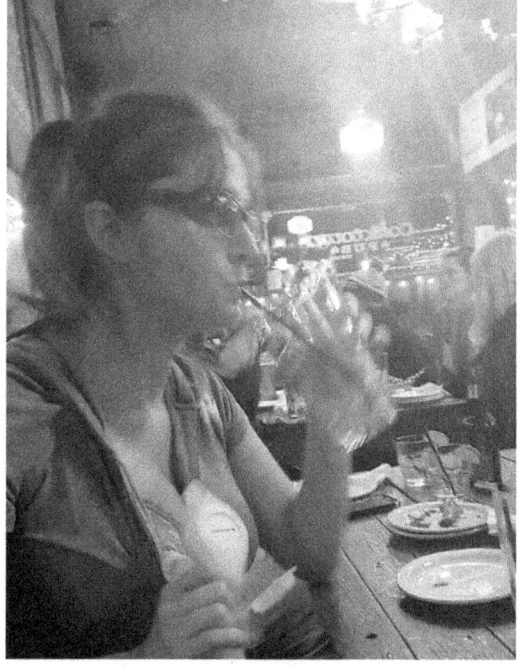

Geoff

Geoff works in Yorkton as I have told you. This year he switched to a new show called Paw Patrol. He is an animator there. He loves it because he has some creative freedom in the scenes. He loves 3D animation work. We are living in a surreal time because each day we enter the store our show is starting to emerge on the shelves. We have no idea at this time how big the show will get. But when at work we are all he can think about. He makes his way here on weekends which is easy enough. But week evenings are tough. It means that he has to take the train back to Yorkton to make it back to work. He tries to come out as much as he can.

We always change into fresh new clothes before coming in, but Geoff prefers to take that extra step of wearing a gown. When Geoff is with Elyot they sing together. Geoff also teaches Elyot to suck on the soothie. It is a very important skill for future eating. Each day Geoff brags that Elyot did three sucks in a row, then later it is ten sucks.

Secondary carers are very important and as I write this book about my experience, I hope more emerge about the supportive people who are not always there but also put in the work.

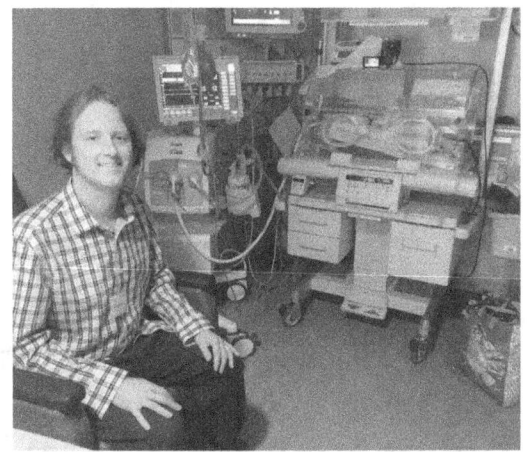

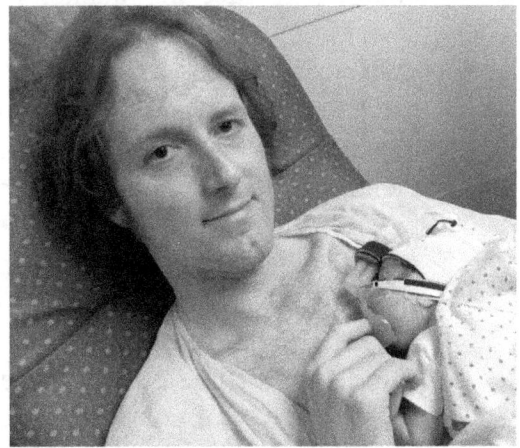

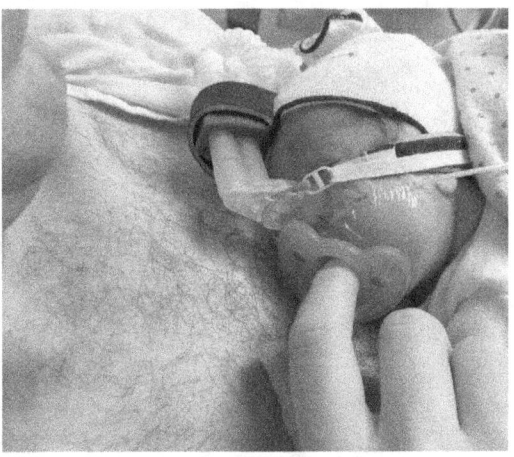

After another weekend of classes, as I walk into the NICU, I see a group of people fussing over Elyot. The monitor is half off. I see Elyot's heart monitor going on and off, trying to fix itself. I see the respiratory therapist there too. I clench my milk to my heart and approach slowly. How bad? How bad? Is this the end? Will there be permanent damage?

"Oh good, mum is here." One of the nurses says. Everyone seems casual and business as usual. I smile and pretend that I am business as usual too and did not just almost have a heart attack thinking something happened. The nurse smiles at me, waiting to tell me the story. I place my milk into the little fridge by his isolette and walk over to this team of professionals. Elyot is full of blood on his face and blanket. It is a scary sight, but if the nurse is smiling, then I should not worry.

She explains that Elyot made his usual Houdini move, freed his hands from the swaddle and went ahead and pulled his breathing tube right out. Houdini is what they call babies who climb out of their swaddles. Elyot has this reputation now, alongside with pulling of his leads and his tubes. He might be a healthier micro-preemie they have here, but he will not let nurses rest during their shifts. There is always an alarm because he pulled something out. Since Elyot has this reputation, the nurse tells me about it in her amused tone. She says it is perfect timing for me to come because he will need to be comforted. He will be a bit unstable for a few hours because intubation stresses him. They return all his leads to the right places, one on the heart, the other two lower on the

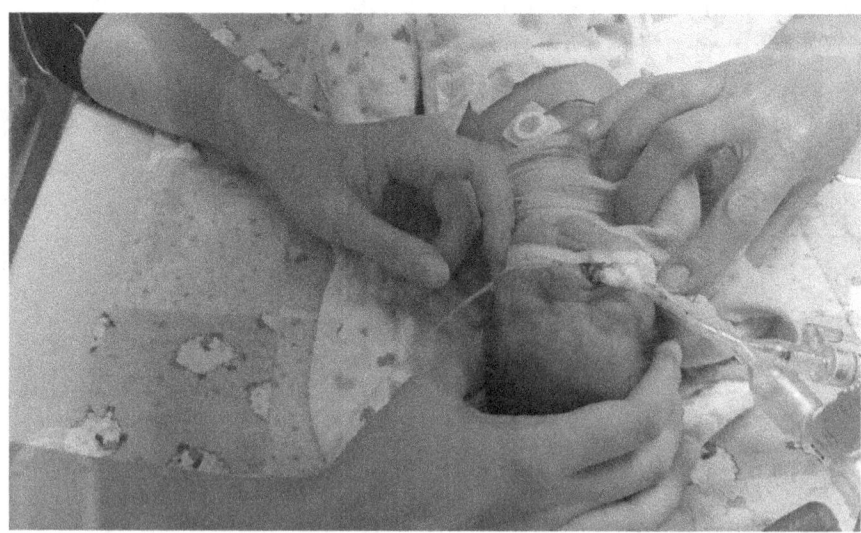

tummy. They wrap another wire around his foot, and the monitor returns to normal. They choose the direction of his ventilator, and now he faces that direction. You cannot turn your face when you are wearing this thing. Whatever direction the therapists decide at that moment is how you lie. His face is still wrinkled in pain. But now he has no more energy to fight us. He has no idea that we are trying to save his life.

Tonight we skip the skin to skin. It breaks my heart because I know how much he loves them, and he has no idea that he just ruined his cuddle with mama. It is these small things that upset me. I look at him, and he is crying with no sound as they finish swaddling him. His lungs are weak on the best days, but currently, he must feel out of breath. His mouth is wide open. He is wincing. It is a huge wrinkly cry but mute. Not a sound besides the monitor being switched back on that is now beeping and sorting itself out.

I place my hands into the isolette and blanket him with my palms. I lower my head. The nurse knows ahead of time and wheels me a chair. I am feeling faint again. For me, this is the first time to see a baby extubate[1] themselves; for her, it is a day at the office. I sit holding him for over an hour till I myself have to leave to pump to the other room. My burning boobs usually tell me when I have to pump. When I return to the NICU, it is their evening shift, and the lights are out. He is soundly asleep because I know the timing of his heart rate when he sleeps. I spend the rest of the evening sitting and watching him.

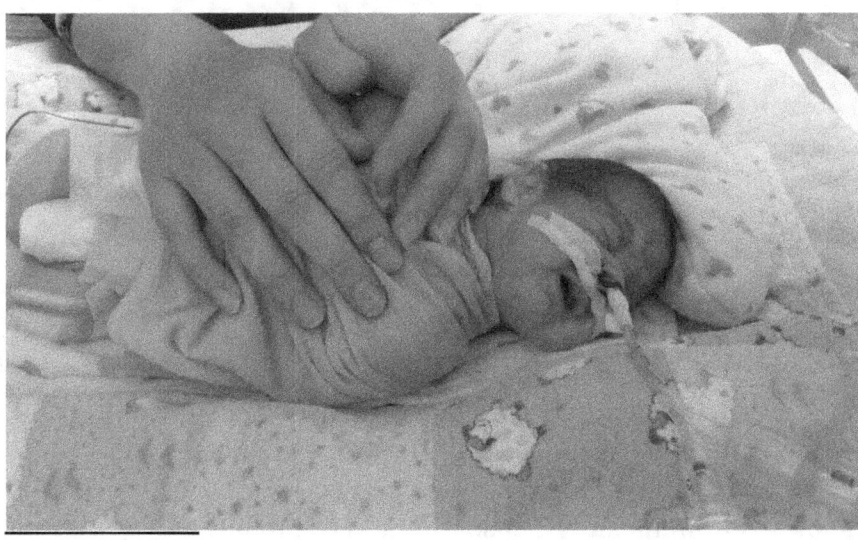

---
1   extubate - to remove the breathing tube

The Machinery

I have had three immigrations, and seven countries that I called home. But I have never been good at languages. Now the NICU has its own language. It talks in through cold numbers, yet the message it delivers cannot be captured by any letters of any vernacular. These numbers tell me stories; they tell me feelings and give me a glimpse into the future. It is an unusual type of language acting as reminders of his birth and an oracle of where he is going. No longer startled by the alarms the monitor sometimes produces, I get to know its subtle eloquence.

His wires are the first interpreter that I get. The wires you see on his first day are called leads. They are attached to three places on his torso area with soft stickers. They are black, white and red and have their placement. At least at my NICU these are the colours.

They measure his vitals such as heart, breathing, temperature and oxygen in the blood. They work at specific parameters, and if those numbers go outside the markers, the alarm goes off. There is also a padded cuff around the wrist that measures his blood pressure. It changes places because the skin is too tender. They rotate wrists and feet so that each limb can rest. Elyot loves removing it and sending off the alarm. They are all a message. They tell me how Elyot feels when I tell him stories, tell me when he is in deep sleep as he cuddles up on my chest, tell me he is growing with the slowing of the heart rate. With time I learn to adjust them. The SAT scores – the finer details of breathing give me worries about his future. Those are a sad song that never seems to end. A melody of how the body takes in oxygen and releases carbon dioxide. I mime kiss them before placing them back into their positions, trying to avoid the red, irritated skin

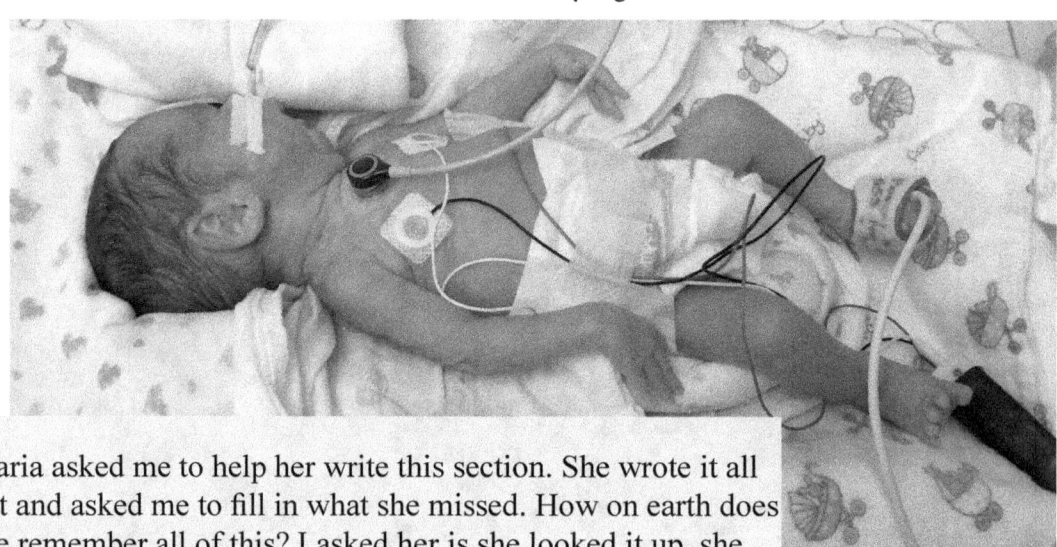

Maria asked me to help her write this section. She wrote it all out and asked me to fill in what she missed. How on earth does she remember all of this? I asked her is she looked it up, she says no, most of it is from memory but some stuff is from his medical notes. I had nothing else to add. She remembered it all. I guess its hard to forget.   *Sasha's perspective*

that held them earlier. A real kiss can happen when he is on me doing skin to skin, and his tiny head is right below my chin. I avoid any risk of transmitting viruses to him. Forgive me if I am so sentimental in a technical equipment section, but these are more than just numbers for us NICU parents.

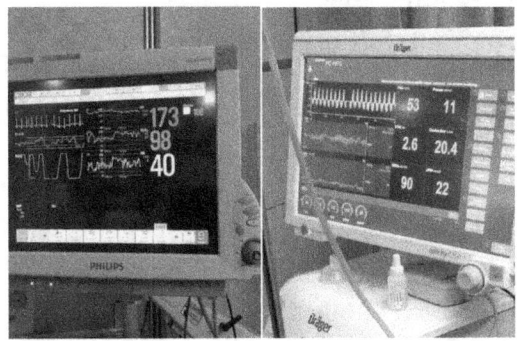

All these lead to the monitor that dominates the room. Those bright colours are the only voice I get from a baby whose lungs are too weak for any utterance.

The second monitor hiding on the sidelines is specifically for the breathing machine. It does not talk to me like the other monitor does but one day when Elyot's breathing is closer to 'room air' I shall become obsessed with it more than a person waiting for election results to come in. Later you get to see this PEEP score. Do not get me started on the drama this thing creates. That PEEP score has to be at '5'. This number means that he can be weaned to a lower oxygen rate. It

If you've been to the NICU, you have a new language. Put that on your resume!

means progress. Everyday you walk in and it jumps around teasing you. If numbers could curse, these ones sure speaks a sailor language!

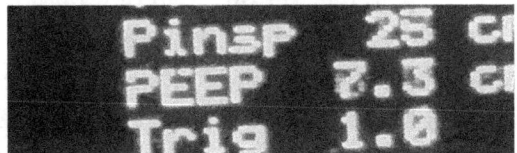

Another gadget that you see standing on a tripod is an automated feeding device. A syringe that measures Elyot's milk feeds and medications and has a slow timed release because the tummy is very sensitive and needs time to adjust. Newborns can drink a whole mouthful, but micro-preemies start with one millilitre and work their way up to bigger feeds. Many babies struggle with feeds. It is not a guaranteed thing here.

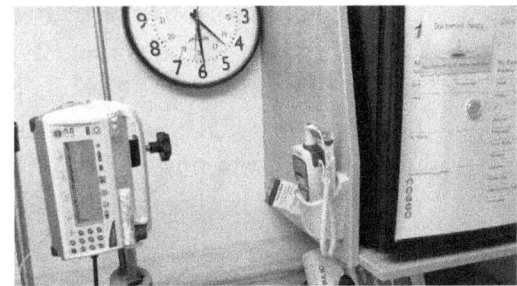

Next to it is a mini-fridge. This is where I place my milk that I bring in. Each baby has its their fridge. They take what they need for today and store the rest. Sometimes you see an IV drip when he has his blood transfusion. His x-rays and ultrasounds are all done here with portable machines.

C PAP Milestone

I am strong enough to walk. My sister works too early so I cannot get lifts from her. Her mother in law Nancy takes me on Fridays. No one else will take me. This morning I make my way there, walking, through the rain. I get such a huge soaker from an ankle-deep puddle. How am I going to spend there rest of the day like this? My plan is to close the curtains, remove my shoe and sock and to hope for the best in the dry NICU air.

My squishy limp leads me to see our hub full of people. This time I am not scared but realize that Elyot must have pulled his tube out again. WRONG! WRONG! Oh glorious puddle had I known this I would have wet both feet with dance and glared into you to see my cheek creasing smile! As if when Elyot pulled off his tube was his last protest, today, he graduates back to a C PAP. He is still on a strong setting where it breaths on his behalf, but now he can work a bit with the machine. His lungs are no longer passive. For us, it means that the last invasive tool is at last out of his body, and his risk of deadly infection has been minimized. Gone are the PICC line and ventilator. But we have been here many times; so we do not celebrate until a few weeks pass because celebrations here are always punished with regressions.

Another win for us is that Elyot can now toss and turn in his sleep, face anywhere he wants because the tube does not chain him anymore. I feel utter joy to know that he is more comfortable now. We get big noses to celebrate. My sister will fetch me later but if I could find that puddle to tell her the good news.

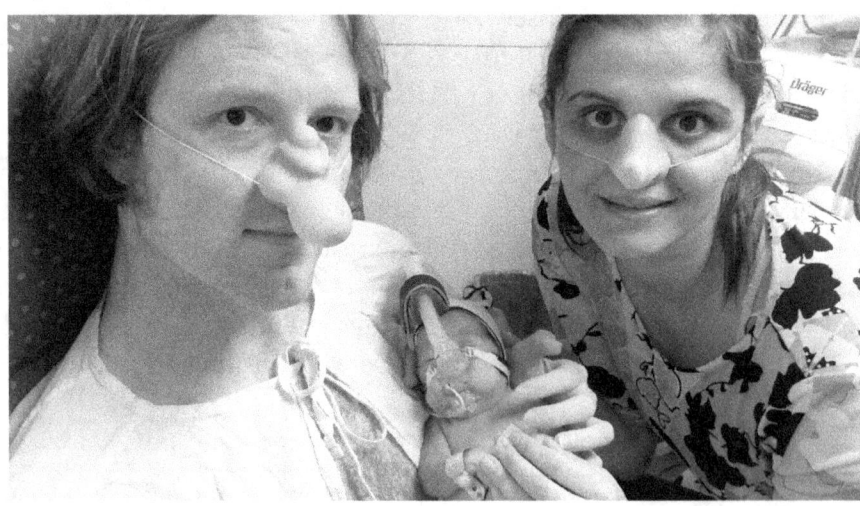

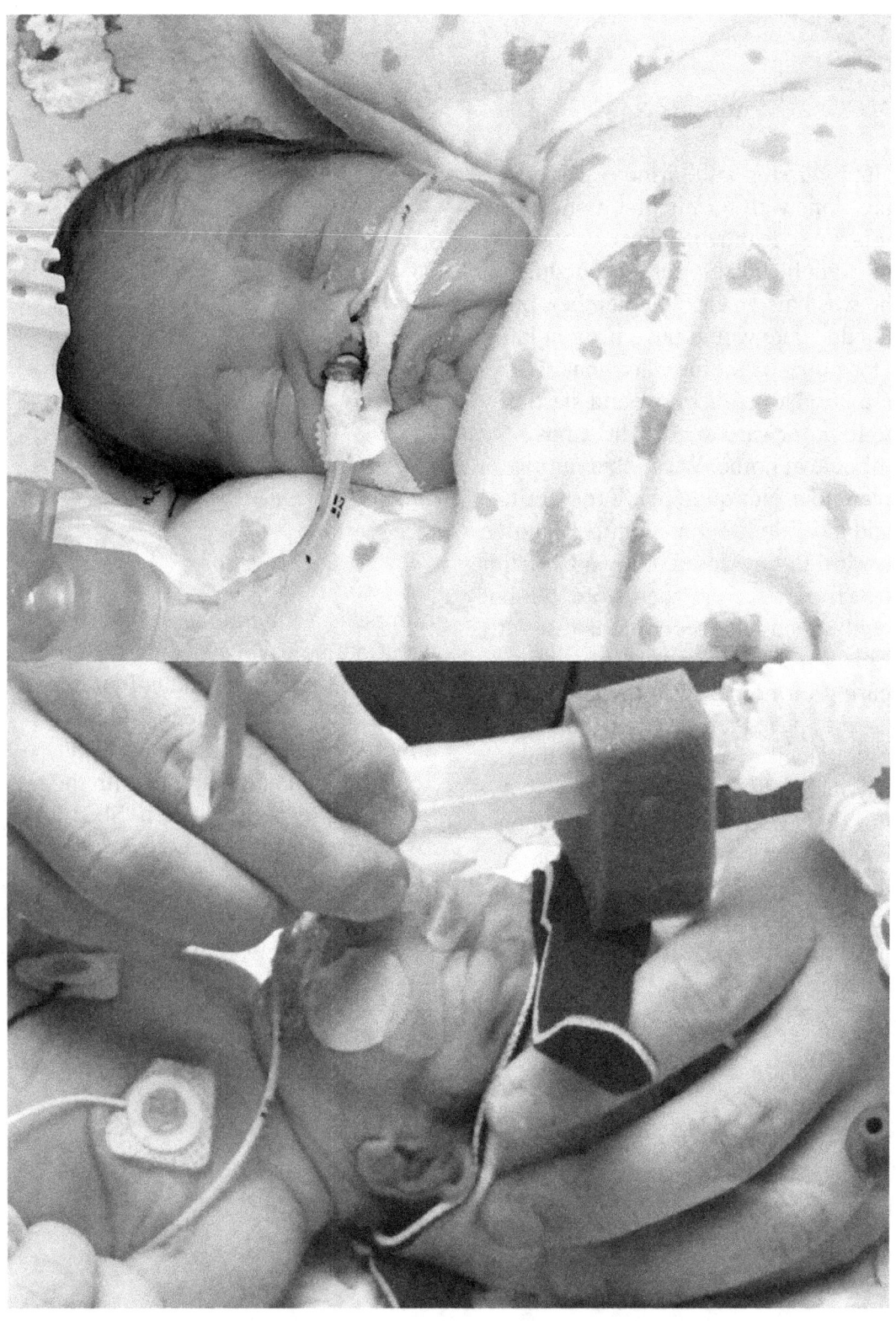

Week 30

Future Is Now!

Happy first month birthday, Elyot! He has done well for his first month, and it is a big deal. No sickness, infections, or brain bleeds. So far on schedule, he was born in early September, but his due date would have been in late December, right for Christmas. We are into November now and starting to look forward to our Christmas miracle at home. We are beginning to plan now. Not quite ready for a crib and a whole life, but slightly planning toward in tiny doses. I buy a Christmas tree from a second hand store, but not ready to buy the decorations just yet. This is a step by step process of preparing for home. Even the good parts need to pace themselves.

Practically speaking , two or three Elyots can fit into a newborn size. A puzzle is what size he shall be when we take him home. He has almost doubled in size, but he is still too small for the tiniest onesie. Will he be a newborn size in December or slightly smaller?

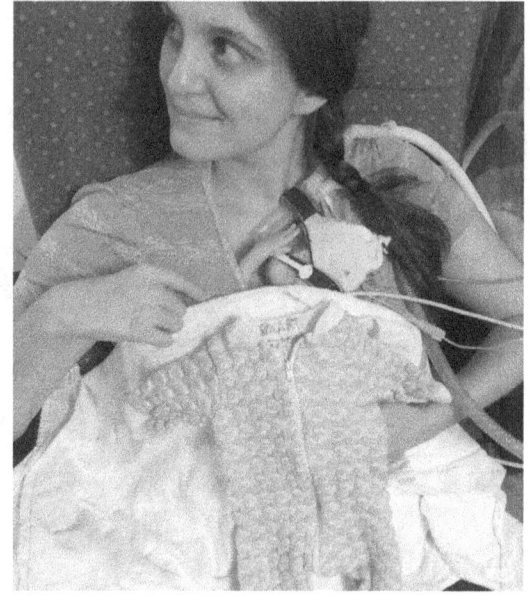

A nurse is asking me which swaddle I want to give Elyot. The one with the pattern on it or this solid colour one. I choose the pattern. She comments on how big he is. I tell her that one day he will be tall and help me with those high shelves in the kitchen. She turns away from me and I feel a very heavy energy push onto us. It seems that I am dreaming too big and too far for her. I thought that its okay to say this after a month here with no complications.

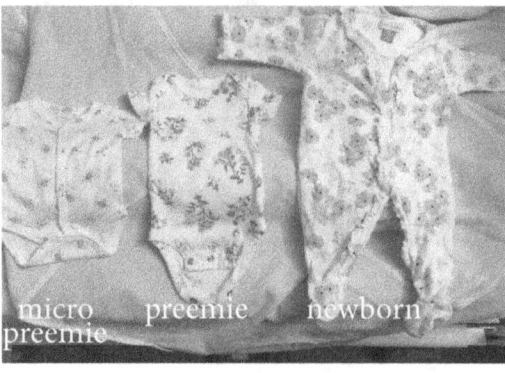

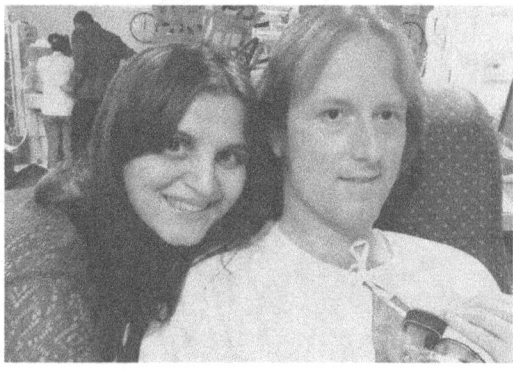

My Pump Routine

My alarm sound is chimes. It is a soft wake up. On my nightstand I have my tablet to watch shows and my pump ready to go. On the dresser close by I have labelled my containers ahead of time so that I have one less thing to do. For night pumping I have a soft night light and but sometimes when I feel sleepier I put on the room light to wake me up. I have soap water in a bowl ready to store my pump pieces that I shall wash and sanitize in the morning. I make sure to have a lot of water next to me because I get thirsty when I pump. I also have close by my nipple cream and heating things in case if I feel engorged. During the day pumps I move my routine to the dining room where I have my computer to watch more shows, eat and do my work.

Sasha's perspective

I see Maria work on a full routine each morning. She takes some sort of vitamins, makes a few teas that she will chub throughout the day and is obsessed with oatmeal cookies and other foods. It is like a science lab here in my kitchen as I see her meticulously setting it up.

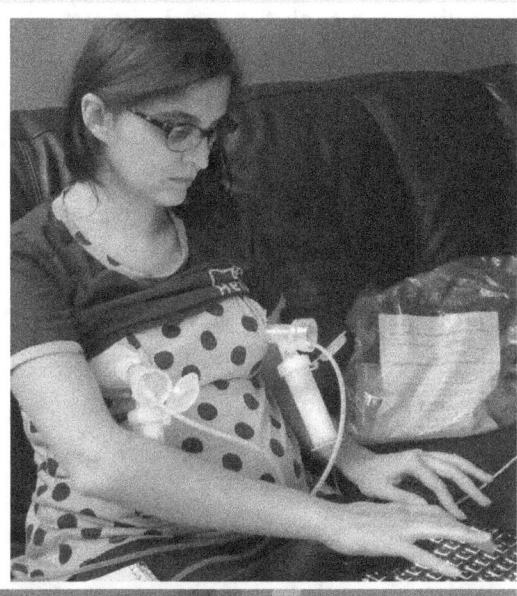

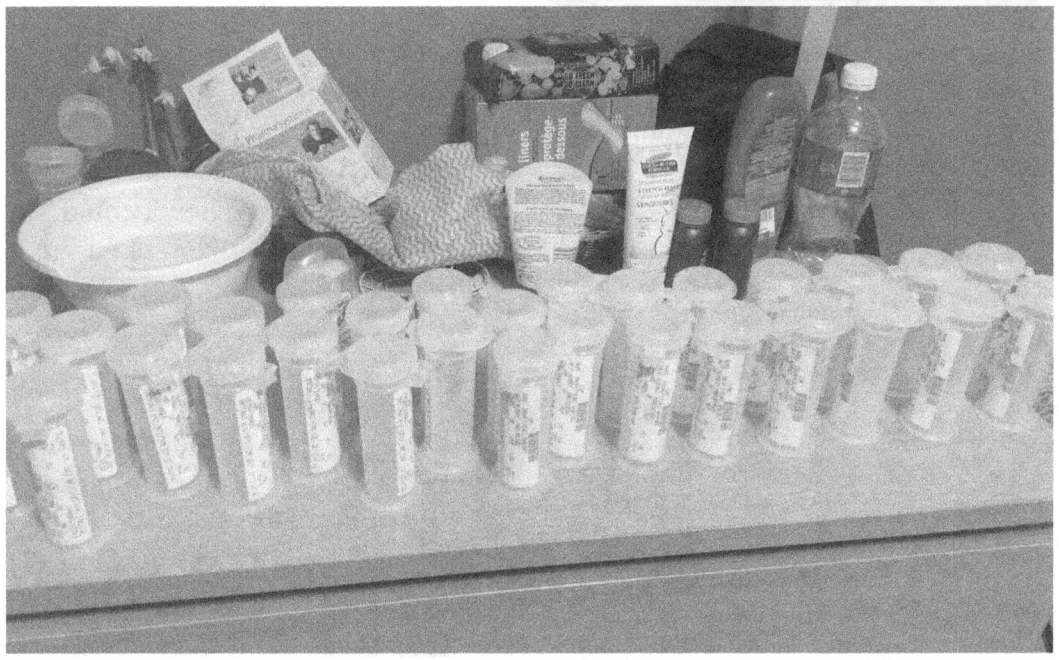

Getting Sick

RVS is the killer of our babies. It means that everyone has to fear you if you have it. If you feel a tiny throat tickle, you're a threat. You cannot visit the NICU and the common area. During these times I ask my sister to deliver the milk for me. I isolate myself from her and everyone to not spread it. I do not ask her to go in on my behalf because I cannot risk her having RSV. Though it is safe to go in if you do not have symptoms, its not worth the risk. At least he will get my milks that day. She does go in my place as I told you when I am in class on the weekends. It feels like a spy mission to get her to go in. Malerie is our main villain. No one notices that she is blonde and already starting to show her pregnancy. Maybe they do notice and say nothing, I have no idea.

Whats the point of having a very similar looking twin if you can't trade places at times? We have done with before when we used a swimming membership. We pretended to be one person to save money. That one was harder because people actually talked to us at the gym. Here no one cares. They leave you alone. I cannot express to you how much I love the people who work here. I have never known such kindness.

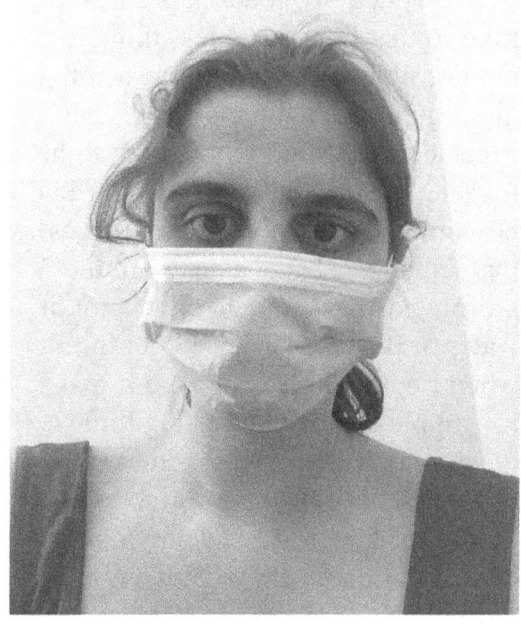

In 2020 when people get Covid 19[1] symptoms, it'll be two weeks isolation. Today thankfully, it can be as short as one day.

Anytime I asked how I could help she'd say "I don't know, I don't need anything." I stopped asked generally and began to offer specific things. "When can I replace you at the NICU? I miss Elyot." "I cooked extra, want some?" "Come with me, I'm going shopping."
Sasha's perspective

---

1   See 126 for more about Covid 19

Week 31

Thanksgiving

Life is now less rushed and urgent, so we become aware of our loneliness and emotional exhaustion. My sister's in laws, the Turples, try to keep us busy as much as they can. Today evening we attend their Thanksgiving meal. It is our first activity outside the hospital since the ordeal started. They are my sister's family but have adopted us as their own in this trying time. Regular parenting needs a village. But when you are a NICU parent, you as the adult need a village too. Outside support is our battery charger. Without them it is very hard to pull through this.

So here we are with his picture open with us as we try to include him. It is emotionally muddled because we have craved this social interaction and relaxation with loved ones, yet being somewhere without our baby is hard. He must be lonely. Someone is usually doing a cuddle with him at this time. We rush back to him the minute we can. He is our home now. We take our celebration to him with plastic decorations since it is the only thing we can sanitize. The nurses are thrilled to see us take this Thanksgiving photo. I think seeing parents get into a celebratory mood makes them happy in this often too sad a place. They, too, are missing this time with their loved ones today.

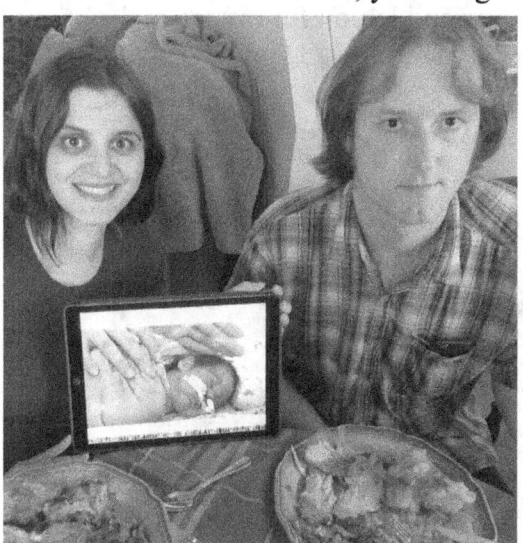

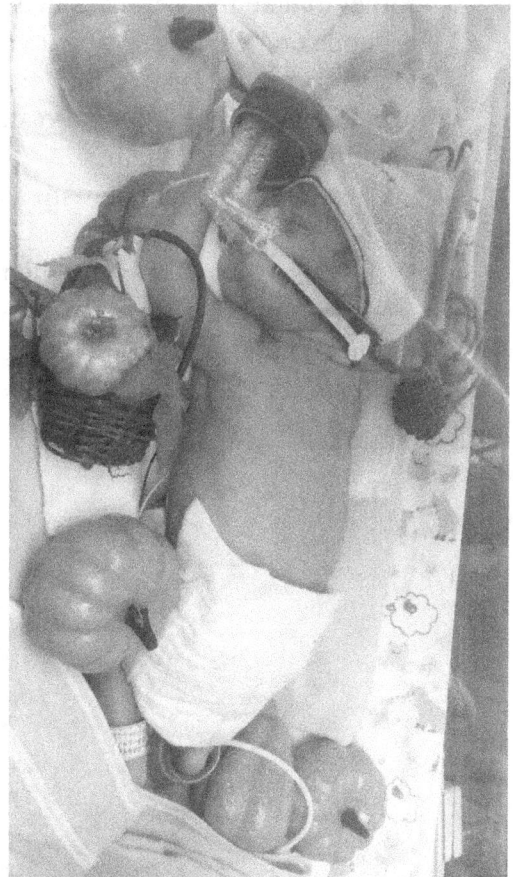

What Is In My NICU bag?

You can always spot a mama with a NICU bag. Somehow its so obvious to us who have been there. The accessory to the giant bag or two that she carries is the posture. Both slow and tired but also excited and in a rush. So what is in mine?

Pump pieces – no need to bring a pump if you NICU provides one in the pump room. Later in Level I bring my own pump to stay by Elyot's side.

Sanitizing things for pumps and to clean your skin to skin arm chair. Some NICUs provide this.

Snacks to secretly eat in the pump room because you have no time to eat. I had cold pizza slices.

Laptop, textbooks, note pad, extra pens for homework that you do while pumping.

Cooler bag with ice packs as you bring in your milks. Don't forget to take more milk containers home as you leave the NICU.

Phone and charger. Bring a very long chord.

If you can be creative like me, I bring a sketch pad and my sketch pencils but end up too sleepy to use them. I bring books to read but never use them.

Camera or your phone with a camera. Clear up space ahead of time.

Onesies if baby can wear them.

What to put into my university bag? All same items but also my pump and do not forget to bring ginger and lemon for my tea and the sharp kitchen knife that is probably not allowed here.

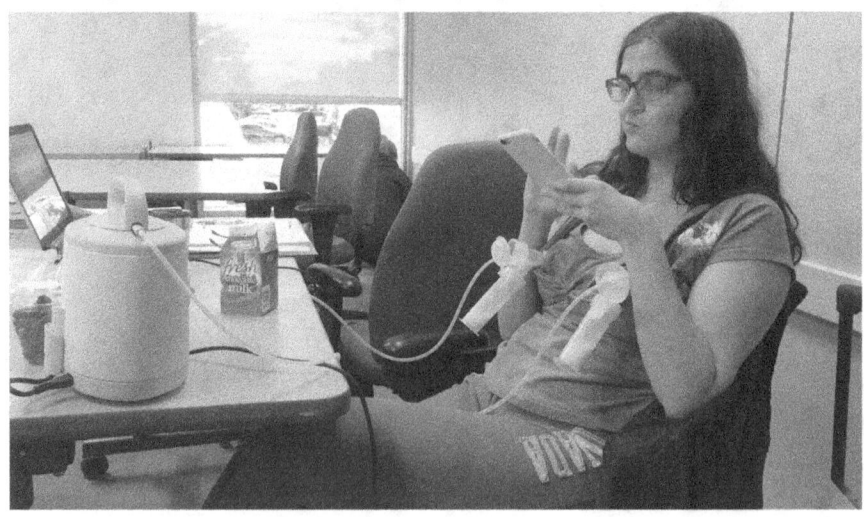

Week 32

Would-Be Born Today

Remember the faded map[1] they gave me in Maternity Ward about all the possibilities of Elyot being born? We have reached the last marker. This is a big week. Week 32 is the week they told me they hoped I would remain pregnant until they would remove him. I would be unable to carry him further with such low fluid. If all worked out in this best scenario today, I would have a baby. He would be on some breathing support still but would not be at risk for any brain bleeds or micro-preemie complications. He would be a just preemie, not a life sentence. I place him under my shirt and imagine the size my belly would have been. It would not have gotten any bigger than this today. I have been robbed of a pregnancy. My dream of walking around looking cute and pregnant. Having bus seats given to me. Wearing maternity clothes. But in return I get to see a secret. I see him develop outside right in front of me. Its beautiful.

I see the fear in her eyes the minute I found out that I am pregnant. She was living with me and I was experiencing first trimester symptoms. She was experiencing pregnancy trauma. One day I had a bad cramp and she found out. The panic that she was trying to hide with her eyes. But then the expression would change. "Micro preemies are not common and I already took that statistic. So you're safe from at least that one." She'd end with a smirk and joke that I need to thank her.
Two sisters with a dark sense of humour. I would not change a thing.
Sasha's perspective

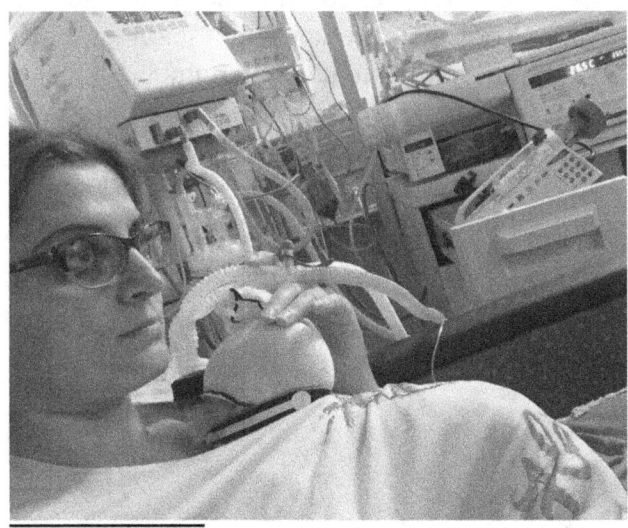
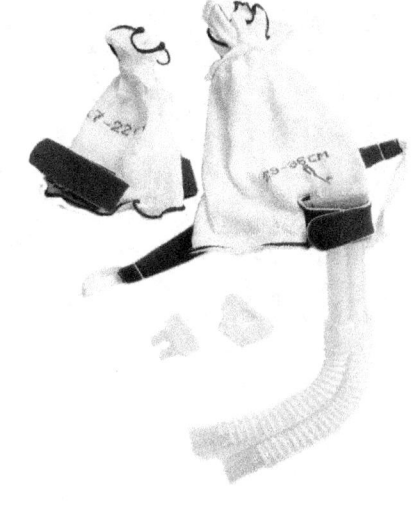

---
1   faded map see pg 15

Eye Test Result

Another significance of this week is that Elyot is scheduled to have his eye test. This day had been on my mind the whole time while other events were happening. The blindness statistic is not mentioned at 26 weeks. But not only was he at 25 but was diagnosed more as 24. I worried about his eyes. Today the doctor finds me and tells me that his eyes are doing well.

His ROP [1] condition is very mild so he is starting off well. It means that his vessels do show signs of stress but at the minimal amount. They will monitor them because oxygen therapy puts them at risk.

When I was in the Maternity Ward thinking about disabilities, I actually was okay with visual impairment, I have friends with it and am not afraid of it. It is a good life if your child gets early support.

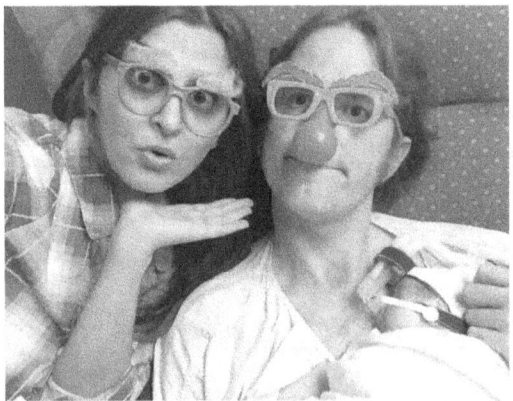

I am sitting with Elyot holding him. An alarm goes off and does not stop. Nurses surround that isolate of that sick baby. His breathing is bad and heart not looking good. This boy has a flu. There is not much anyone can do but hope that he overcomes it. More nurses gather as the alarm refuses to subside. I see the urgency in everyone watching. Come on buddy you can do it! Please buddy! Come on! Pull through. Some are praying, some are swaying with stress. It is so tense right now as I hold Elyot closer to my chest. I close my eyes and think of his mother who is not here and unaware.

Finally red numbers are yellow, then green and the alarm is gone. He has stabilized. Nurses take their deep breathes of relief and without word they resume their stations. They continue their work as if nothing happened. They must be used to this. I am shaking in residual fear. I just witnessed how much these nurses care about our children when we are not here. This mother might learn later that her baby fluctuated in numbers but she might never know the crowd of nurses who cheered her baby back to life. This boy will get better and will go home eventually but meanwhile today is fighting for his life.

---

1 ROP- Retinopathy of Prematurity. See pg 21

New Activities

To add to our parenting roles this week, they teach us how to bath him with all the tubes. They place him on the table with a warm wet washcloth. He cries, of course. His skin is still tender.

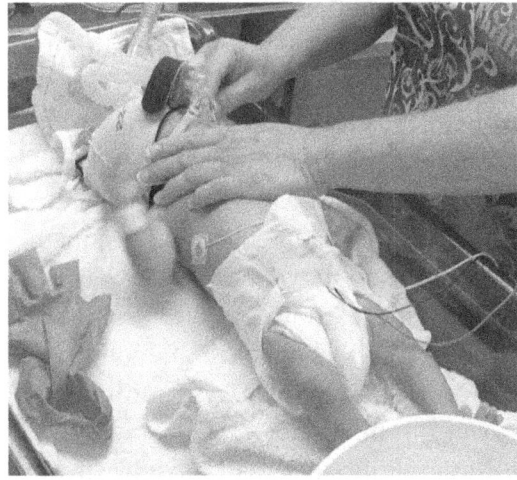

We also start to teach him to take food orally by putting a cue tip in his mouth with milk. He loves it—his first actual taste of food. Today are licks. One day he will eat.

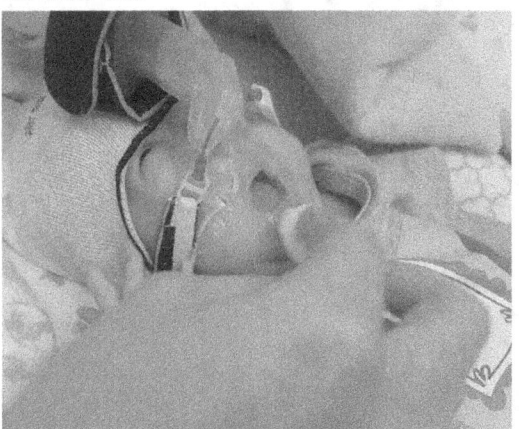

His oral muscles are stronger, and his mouth is bigger to he graduates to the bigger preemie soother. It is huge on him because he is still tiny. He often falls asleep trying to suck on the soother, but we keep working on his stamina. His oral muscles and lungs and breathing all work together to suck.

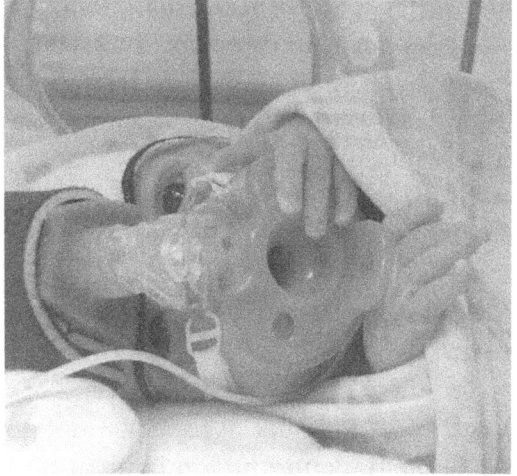

Since micro-preemies are not common, we participate in many scientific studies. I am happy to help future babies, so I sign him up for all of them.

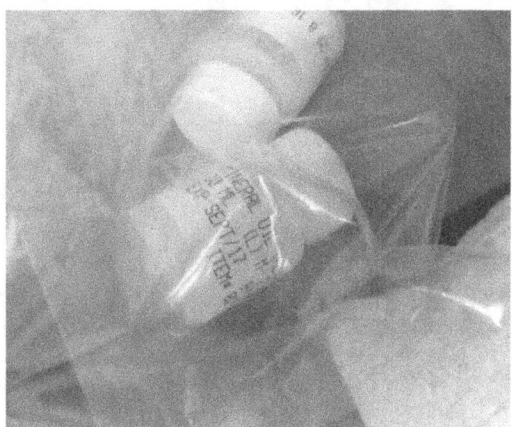

Bad News About His Lung

This week started well but ends completely devastating. We have our routine follow-up with the doctor. All the attention draws to Elyot's lungs. They are struggling to wean his C PAP. He is stuck at PEEP 12; they want it at 5 with oxygen of room air at 21. Alien language to mere observers, but fellow NICU parents will understand. That PEEP has been the same number for a while, and I did not know that it meant anything before today. Long story short, but why is he not improving? Worry sets in. They attempted to lower his need for oxygen, but he is not ready.

He is now on the most severe end of the chronic lung disease spectrum. I do recall them mentioning inflammation and dryness a lot in doctor's rounds. Now am told that his lungs are succumbing to his micro preemie origins. His low fluid month when he was in the tummy adds to the lung distress. The doctor explains that other lungs are like a balloon; Elyot's is more like a paper bag. I taste vomit in my mouth hearing that. Our fighter can do it no more. His marathon has been run out, and he is out of breath just existing. They tell me that he will need to be on oxygen when he goes home and that this will be his problem for the rest of his life. It will not be severe, but not to expect him to win in the Olympics. I shall never tell Elyot that the doctor told me this, and if he wants to train for the Olympics one day, I will support him. Another prediction is that Elyot will also be sicker than other children and have a lower immune system in his life.

Meanwhile, they will have to slow down all his breathing therapies because they are hurting him and causing stress to his already inflamed lungs.

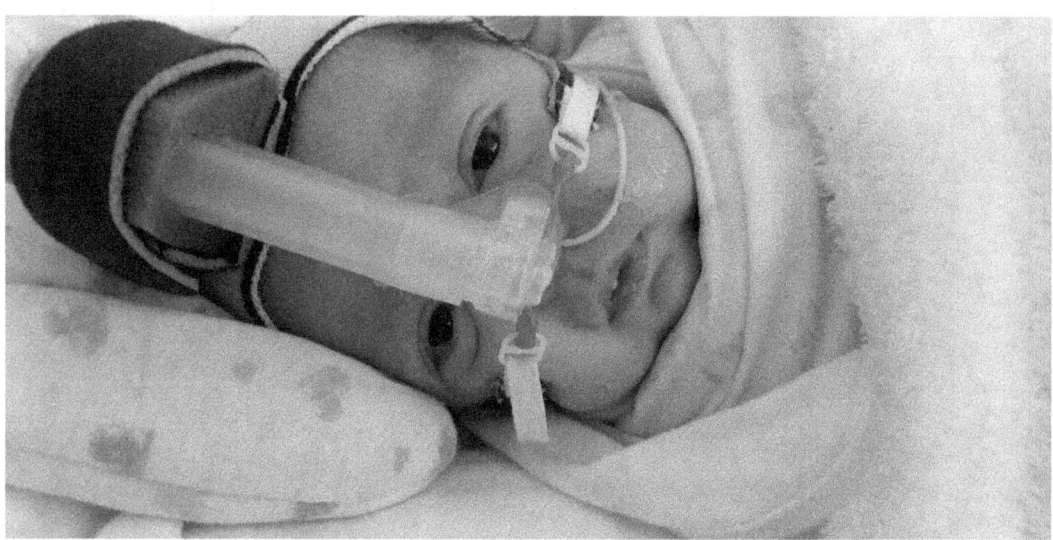

They will slow it to stop anymore damage from occurring until he grows bigger and fatter. To grow bigger is one of the most painful things a doctor can say because no one grows bigger overnight; it is another way of saying that this will take a while. To fatten him up, they decide to add some calories into his milk.

This session ends with the harsh truth that Elyot is not coming home for Christmas. He will not be a cute decorative piece lying next to the tree I just bought at a second-hand store. We will not be a family sipping hot chocolate together, happy to finally be home as we watch him sleep by a frosted winter window. Not us. His lungs are severe such and such. The following day, they decide to give him another blood transfusion to help his blood carry oxygen around. Elyot has still not caught up to do this on his own. There hangs a little blood sac next to him. Besides the colour, it does not look different from anything that has a slow drip and timer. Is he aware of what is happening? He is deep in his sleep. His heart is slow.

Later as I leave to pump and return, I see him with a tiny bandage on his hand. He is exhausted, little hands out of his swaddle but too tired to fully climb out as the usual scene when I come in.

Even little Houdini couldn't make it fully out of the blanket. No cuddles today because he is too tired to be taken out. Elyot won't miss my heart music today anyways. He is too far somewhere else as new tourist blood makes its way through his little body. I don't cry. I weep

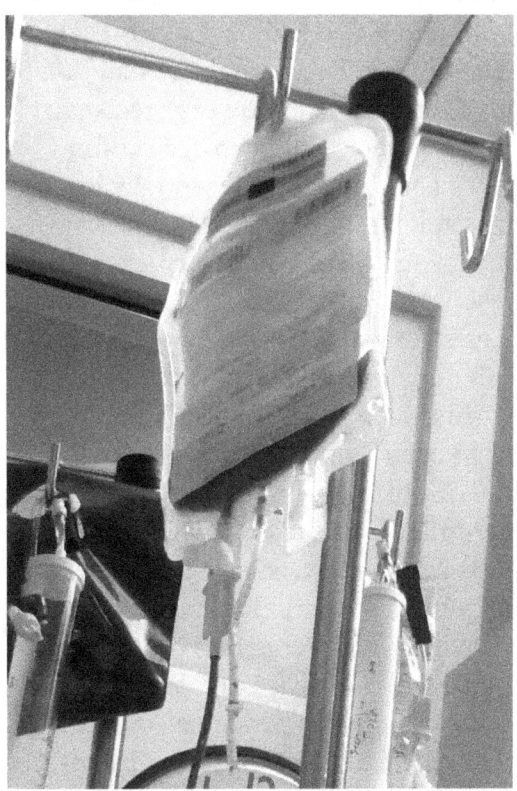

I weep for Elyot. I choke on tears of isolation. I wail for non-stop pumping that sees no breaks, no weekends. I scream because no one understands me. I cry because I hide my tears. My face a turbulent storm.

Week 33

Donation Time

The NICU is a boat going against the stream. It is exhausting and emotionally taxing, but you have no choice but to keep the steady row. There is no option to let go and drown. You cannot take breaks. You cannot say that you give up. The boat, however resistant to the stream, still keeps going forward against your will. You decide how, though. Either you just survive it, or you pull at your every strength resource. The way to do it is to find battles to win. That is your gas, your solar energy, your steam.

This week I finalize a side battle I have been working on for a while. I finalize the process to donate most of my milk. It was tedious with blood tests and doctor visits. It took weeks to prove that my milk is clean for them. Now I have my donation baggies, and I measure out what I am donating. Today a delivery person is coming to fetch them all. However low I might feel, this is a huge battle I just won and a wonderful distraction.

I have a purpose now. Elyot is only feeding a tiny amount but I am producing a lot. To save other sick or premature babies and to bail out struggling parents who cannot produce milk. However hard their boat ride is, I hope my milk will ease their stress.

The amount that I counted at home is 50 litres worth; I think the NICU has more than that amount. It is a risk that if my milk suddenly stops, I have donated all my previous milk. But to keep it is to waste it because it has a shelf life and others need it urgently. The risk is worth it. Today I am so happy.

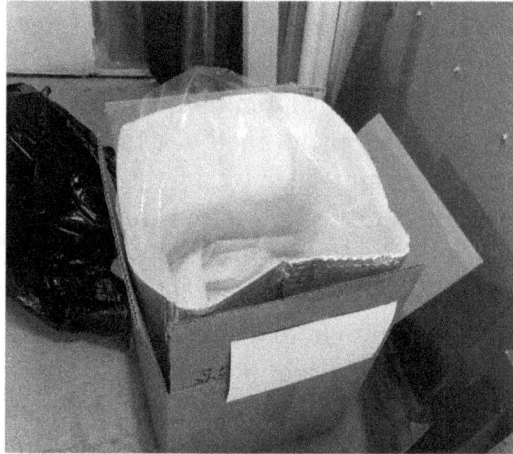

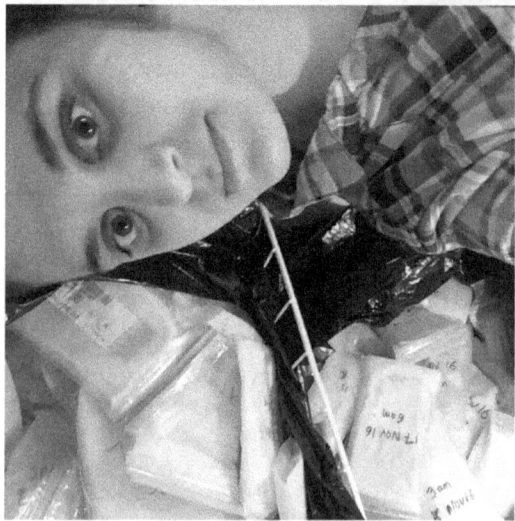

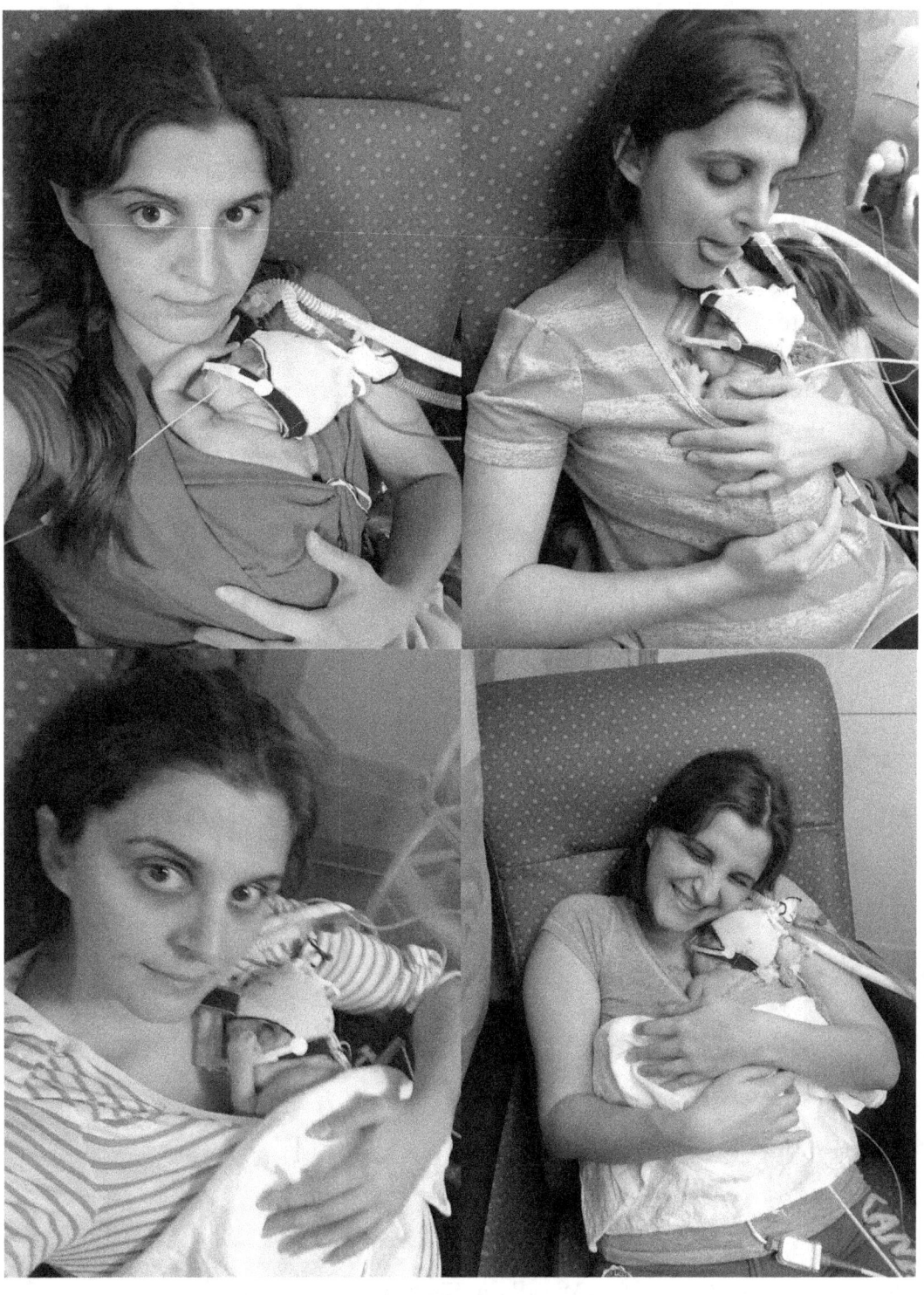

Sometimes when I am alone at my sister's house I feel free to cry my lungs out. Not a timid hidden cry that usually happens in bed , but a loud one where I am on my knees on the floor. I am not depressed. I do not think I am. If there is such a thing as a pump depression, then maybe I have that one.

Later I look at the time and realize that my sister will be home soon. I need to hide my face. Wow look at this face staring back at me in the mirror. It is swollen. No amount of make-up can hide this.

I do not wear make up. I am a simple person. However during this NICU time I start to wear it. I try to hide my spirit from the world. I wish there was make up for my soul, not only my face. Do I even still have a spirit?

What is a spirit?

Once I see my Elyot I forget why I ever cried. He makes me love life again.

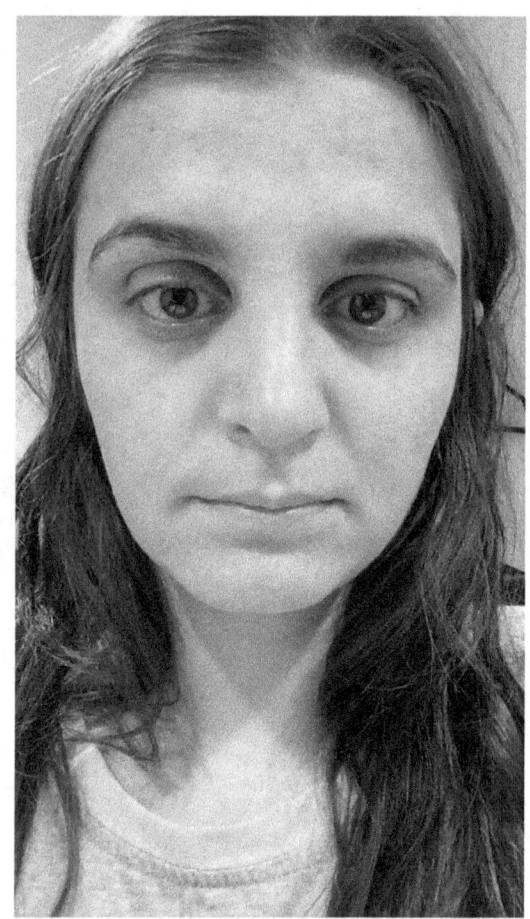

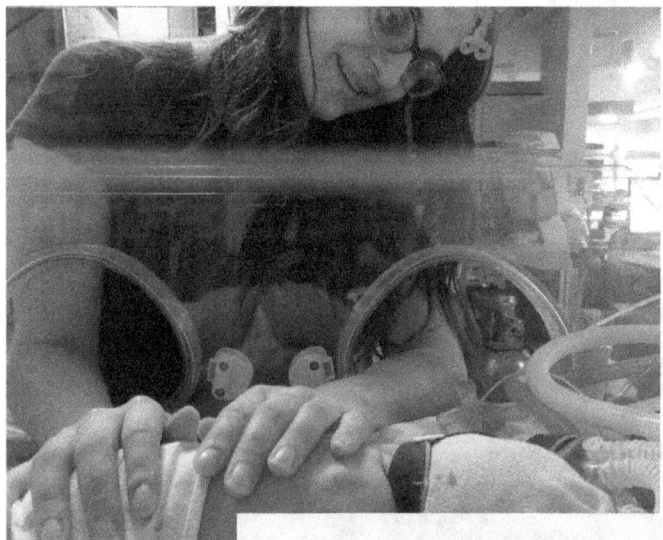

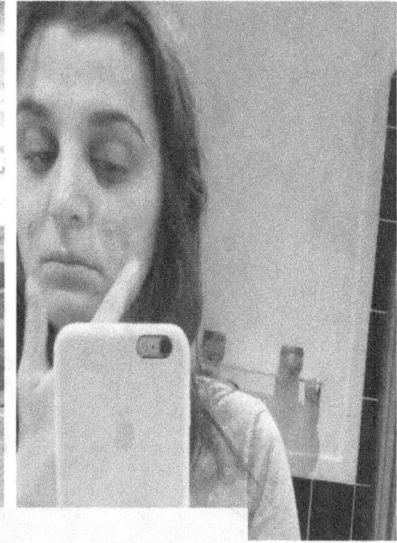

I do notice. We all do. Your face gets swollen, red, and you intentionally put hair over your face. I just play along because I know you. On my end I hide my own puffy face from you. We try to find ways to distract you. To not give you time to cry.

Sasha's perspective

Onesie Milestone

The boat continues moving forward, and we enjoy the tiny things. They are not always medical celebrations but today Elyot is wearing a onesie. It means that his body can now regulate his own temperature, so that he can now wear clothes. It means that they might put him into the crib soon. Isolettes are there to create a temperature for the baby who cannot do it themselves. It is time to go shopping for premature-sized clothing! What a dream! They only sell preemie clothing in stores, micro preemie only exists in specialized stores or for dolls. We cannot afford those, so what we bring in shall be baggy on him for the next while. But it also gives us another lovely responsibility – to dress him. Photo: We wear pyjamas too, to celebrate Elyot's onesie. This one was strange to explain to the nurse why we are in pyjamas.

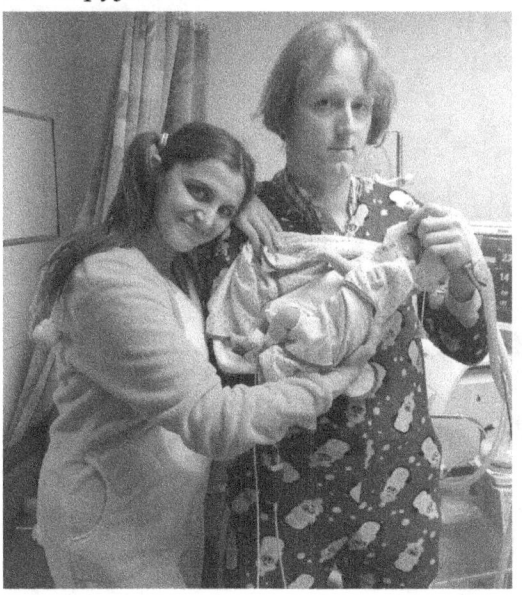

Halloween Costumes

What on earth can you do with a baby at the NICU attached to tubes and wires? At this point, we are no longer asking for permission to bring costumes. Elyot is stable enough, and parents are encouraged to become independent here. He is a hybrid of Geoff and me, who are different bugs. A bumblebee and a ladybug.

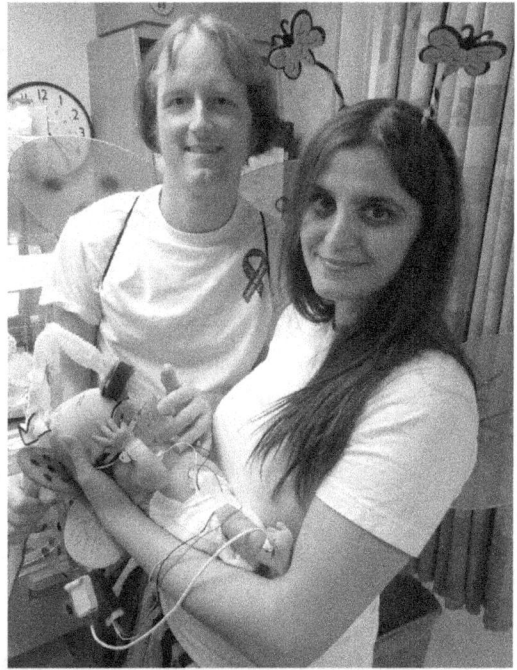

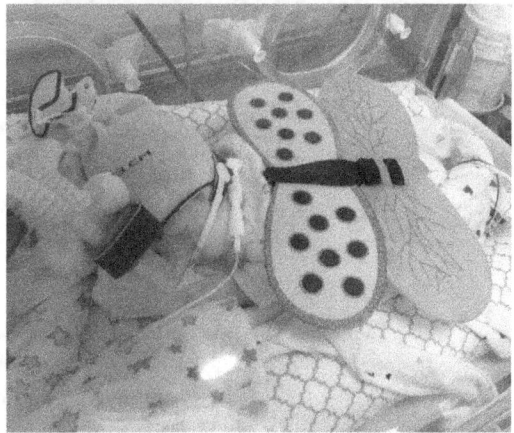

Geoff walks into the NICU as he does any other day. With flutters in his heart to approaches Elyot's isolette. It is extra foggy looking today, harder to see inside. Yes something is off right away. He focuses his eyes to figure out what is wrong. What happened to Elyot?

He is looking exhausted, all limbs are lying flat on the sides. His skin is different, more crimson. What happened to his chubby pink look? What is worse is that Elyot also shrunk in size. How does a baby shrink?

Geoff stares at his sick baby. All gains have been lost. What does this mean for Elyot? Does Maria know about this? A sickening feeling enters him. Is this normal? Maybe babies have a certain growth then they shrink a bit before they can grow bigger? Is this natural? Or is this bad news today?

"Who are you?" A nurse overseeing this hub asks.

" I'm papa Zak, Elyot's daddy. What happened here?"

"That's not Elyot."

"Huh?"

"Who is Elyot? Oh wait, they moved a baby this morning from here. I think you daddy are in the wrong place." Nurse gives a wink. She motions for Geoff to follow her and leads him into another pod.

"There he is."

And indeed there he is! His same chubby cheeks, arms playing with the air. Big C PAP hat. He has been moved to a slightly less urgent part of the Ward and replaced by what I think is a newborn probably in its 30's gestation-wise but frail because it was just born.

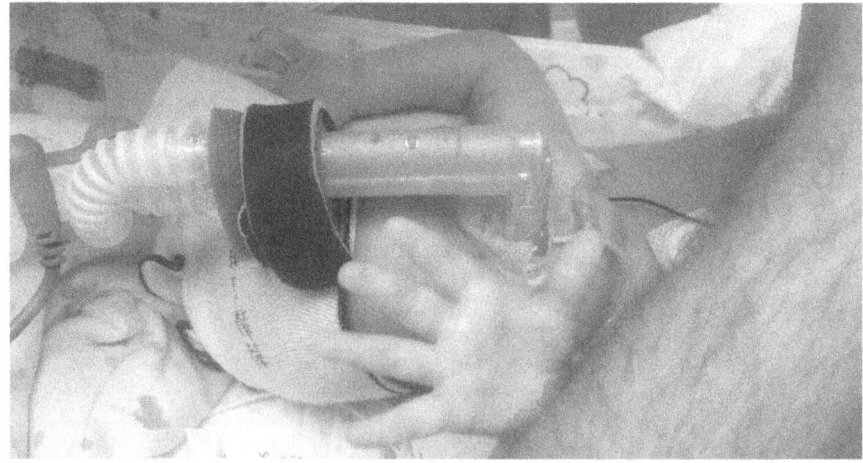

Week 34

Two Month Anniversary

If born today, Elyot would breath on his own. He would lie in the isolette for a few days with jaundice, and we would spend a couple of weeks teaching him to feed. After that, unless there are other health issues, Elyot might go home early and super tiny, according to different babies I have seen here with this gestation.

This month is not exciting as the first month was. Actually is rather routine. Elyot's lungs are nowhere near coming off oxygen as they work on fattening him up. He might have oxygen at home or a tracheotomy. Also, they tell us they might need a G tube[1] if oxygen gets in the way of him learning to drink milk. All the wins and gains are slowed down, and we are struggling again. So tired.

I miss my parents. Gosh, I need my parents. For papa to play on the guitar and mama to dance, brother to make jokes, as we always do together.

Legally Alive

This week we legally register Elyot as a newborn. I was afraid to do this before and thought it might jinx his life if I did it too early. But with the risk of infections mostly gone and the only main issue is his lungs, we know that we are eventually taking him home. I press on the box "NO" where the question asks if the subject is deceased. I cry because I am happy, but I also cry because of my friends who birthed stillborn angels. There is no truly happy place filling this out when you have seen tragedy in other lives.

That is why you will not hear me refer to Elyot as a miracle baby. I refuse to receive a miracle if other parents do not get one. It is not fair. Not a miracle but a winning ticket in the gamble of life. I lost the pregnancy lottery but I hit the jackpot in the micro preemie game.

Today Elyot exists in the computer. He is legally alive.

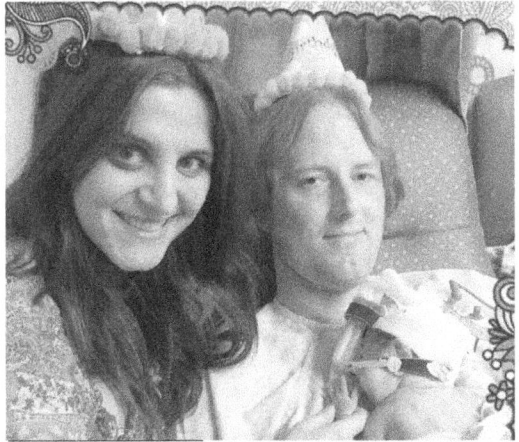

[1] G tube is a feeding tube inserted into the baby's tummy because they cannot feed orally.

Not Compromising Expectations

I have a 25 weeker baby at the NICU. Baby was born over 3 months premature. I'm very lucky that it is not less than 25 they say. I am lucky that my baby had a good brain ultrasound. I am lucky that my baby ONLY has a severe lung thing. Very lucky! He is growing bigger and fatter. He pooped soon after birth. VERY LUCKY. I have to be grateful! So what if they are adding weeks to his discharge. I am so fortunate that he is otherwise healthy.

They say.

They act as if I chose this NICU experience and now I have to deal with compromises since now I am here. But why cannot they understand that I do not want ANY of these health challenges? Why do I have to be strong and to be happy with whatever is handed to me --- because it can be so much worse.

I do not want any of this. I am upset at every regression. I am devastated that every talk of development that ends in " but he's a micro preemie" "amazing for a micro preemie" "miracle baby, you are so lucky since he's a ...you know.....a micr-

Dear doctor, nurse, health person at NICU, friend, family member. How about I decide when I am lucky. How about I decide when miracle talk is appropriate. Why do I have to contend with your compromises just because you expected the worse? I want the best and it is my right to feel that way. But you keep wanting me to count my blessings.

I sigh. My sigh is a long gust of wind. I just want a healthy full term newborn. Not to worry about his future cognitive development, or his immune system. And you are making me feel horrible for wanting what others have, for wanting what was promised to me.

I rub my laboured brow. How do I phrase it in a way you can understand me?

Perhaps one day I shall come on here and write a blog about how blessed I am regardless of all the challenges my baby has, but that is my decision to do that, not yours. It is my decision to overcome this.

Yes I acknowledge that my baby has it better - for a micro, but I want it all to be great. I do not want him to suffer. I want him back in my tummy where I can protect him. As a mother I want the best for my child.

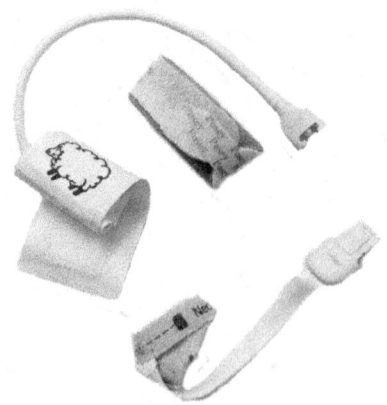

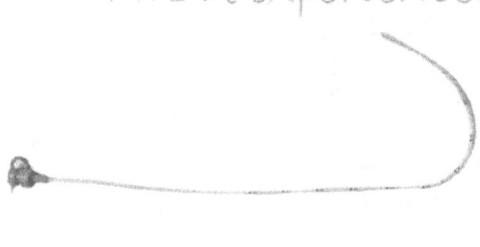

I did not choose this NICU experience.

Week 35

Fat

What I thought will take months takes a week. When a baby is so small, calories make a huge difference very fast. Their plan was to put his lungs on hold with weaning oxygen therapy till he got stronger to deal with it. Talk about fat! This is a different baby. Who is this? From a frail skinny thing, he turned into a goofy teddy bear. I am interacting with two other micro preemie mothers, and their babies are not tolerating anything in their digestive systems, and those babies need surgeries. I understand the importance of tolerance and that Elyot has a great stomach for this. I appreciate it, and we celebrate it as with anything else.
FAT!

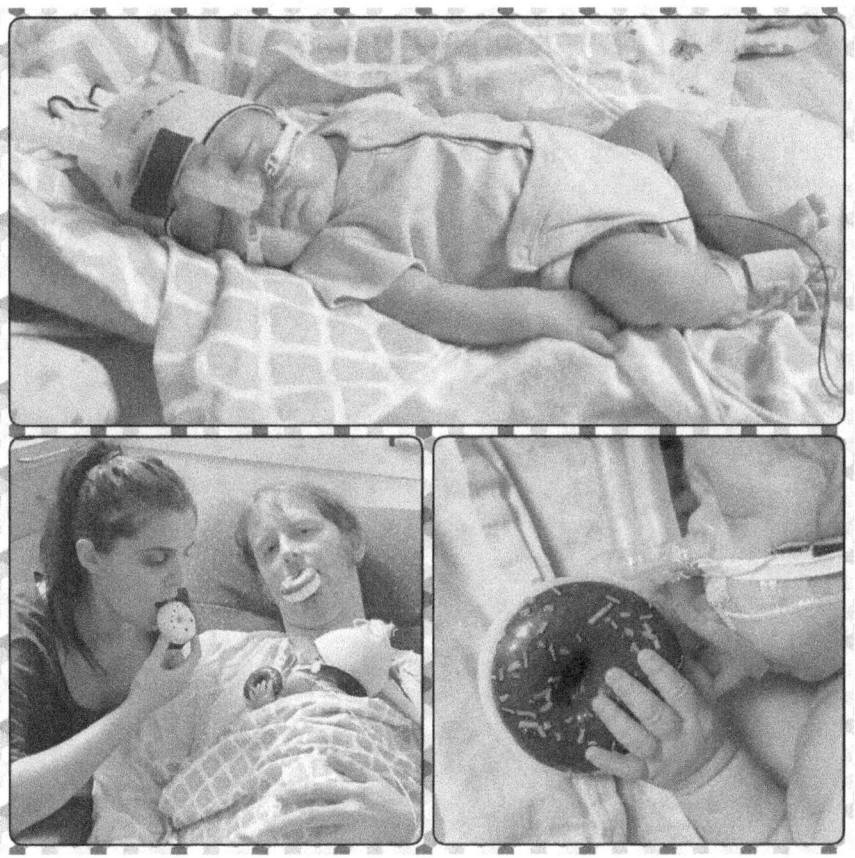

Another Vacancy

Another baby has gone home. We are still here. The only mobility we get is changing hubs within the ward. Seeing another empty space reminds me how long we are here. It is a slow cooking sadness. When in Maternity Ward, time was physical, in this ward; it is still. Nothing moves in your world, but the outside passes by without looking at you. Horrors arise from across the world. I hold onto Elyot tightly as I hear ISIS emerging across the globe. Whether it is routine or world politics, I witness staff here practicing and discussing emergency evacuation procedures. Perhaps these were always there, but I notice a lot of code announcements. Code White or Code Blue. I am hyper aware. Its a topic for another book but I am a child of war and have trauma related to this. It is a very nervous time for me and even the alarm sounds startle me again.

We do not unpack the Christmas tree because we are not going home then. I do not feel any joy in these events but rather heartbreak at what was taken from me. The following day, that empty space is occupied by another baby. Another family gets the viability chat from the nurse and my weeping is back for that child as I follow its alarms and doctors' rounds messaging about its health. Another baby, another empathy attack.

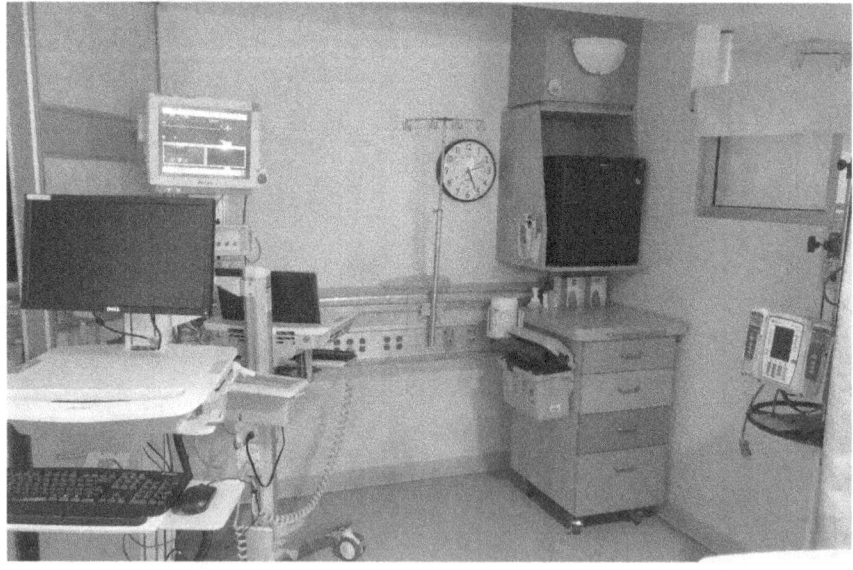

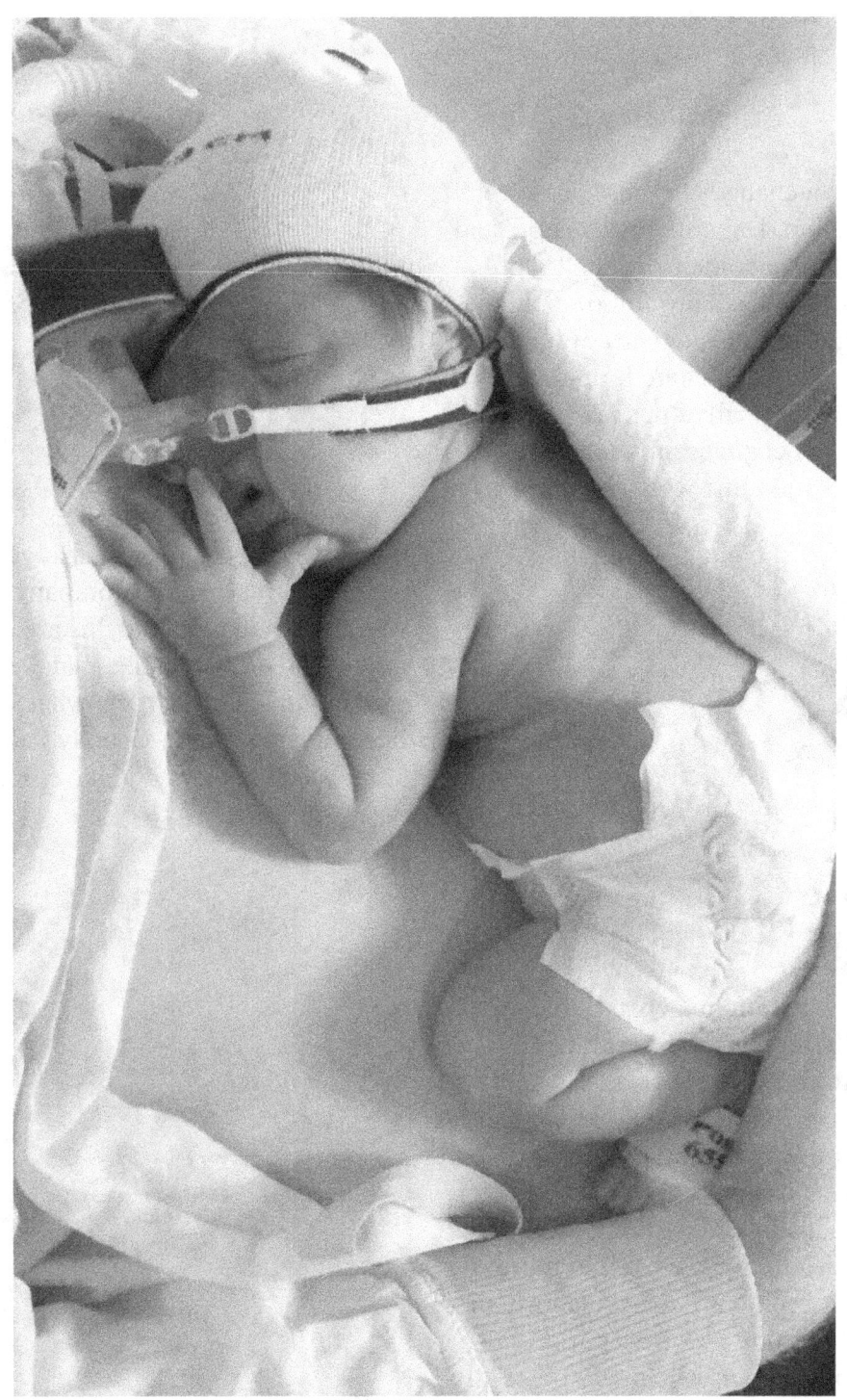

Week 36

⭐ Crib Milestone

Not much changes in these last weeks of gestation. Days seem the same, and I do not have home to which to look forward. My days are full of cuddles, reading, drawing sketches of him and singing. I try to change it up for my sanity. One usually does not get a warning of changes at his isolette corner; one often just walks in to discover it.

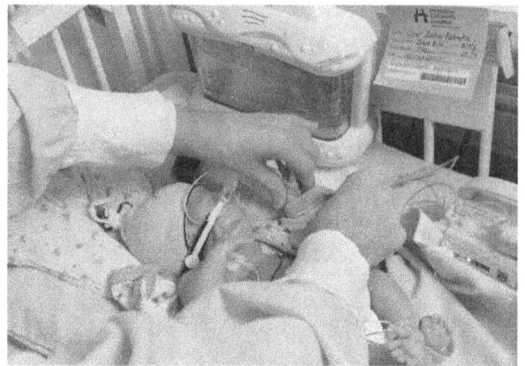

I cry happy tears today. With no glass between us, he can look at us now when we talk to him. He also gets an aquarium to keep him company. Only when small details like this are added to our hub do we realize that we were missing this. One forgets what it is like outside of here. Usually babies at home sleep in cribs and have things to entertain them.

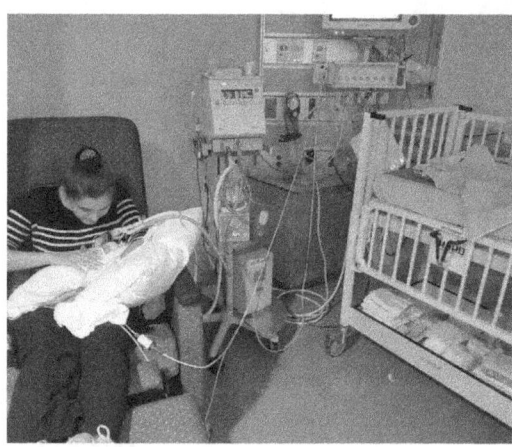

Today I see him in a crib. Babies who can fully regulate their body temperature can sleep in cribs. He could handle a crib weeks ago, but we had to wait for one to become available. He is now exposed to outside viruses, so we schedule an RVS shot, as this virus can be deadly for micros. No more glass between our two selves, just air between us now! Warm sanitized air! To embrace your little one. Forget all the mean numbers on the monitors. This is bliss. Nothing else matters!

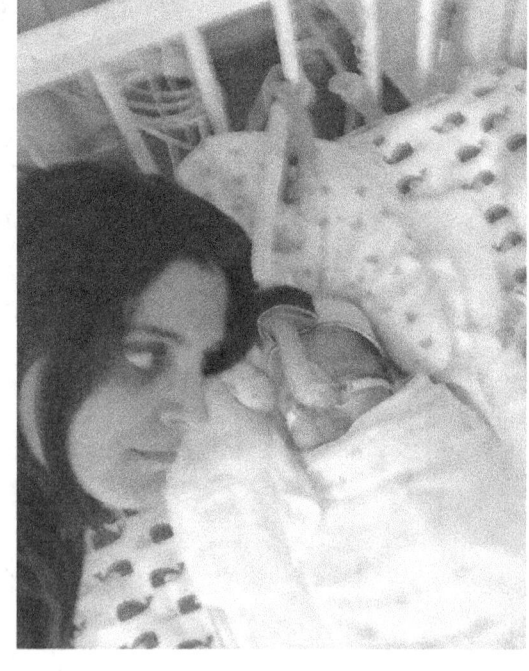

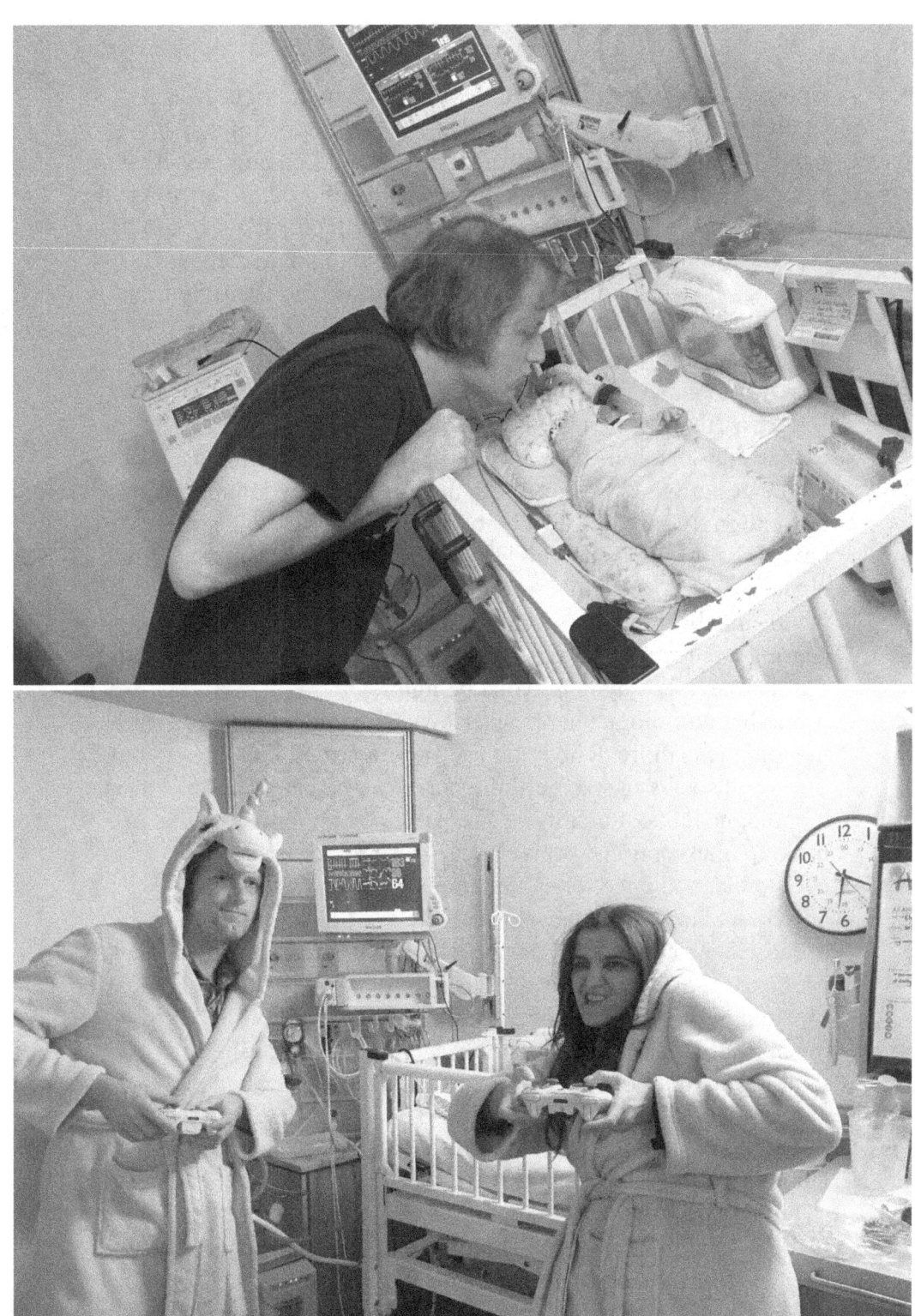

NICU Monologues

Another monologue. Call it a NICU nurse's monologue. See her sit on a black stage beneath the sizzling warm glow of a spotlight. she sits straddled backwards on a chair. Leaning the elbows against its back. She is rough in her gentleness. Like crunchy cereal in milk. She tries to be slow, maternal, affirming, but to them she sounds like a rock.I turn my head to the audience. Depending on the monologue script I can guess who is sitting in the audience.

Today's monologue is about the RSV virus. A disease barely noticed by many adults but can be fatal for premature babies. Bigger premature babies who are outside isolettes are at risk. Its like a flu that kills. I guess that the baby across me must be of late gestation. It was just born and already they talking about prevention. It took longer than two months for me to get this talk, but this baby across the pod is having it already on first day. The nurse is cold as she explains the dangers of RSV. She recommends that baby get a preventative shot. I feel sorry for the parent hearing this lecture but also I envy her that her baby gets this talk on day one. Her stay here won't be long.

Another monologue happens elsewhere on another stage. This monologue is more deliberate, each word treated like fine crystal. The stage swells in size until the nurse can be barely visible. This monologue talks of quality of life, talks of no promises, talks of back up interventions, I raise to my feet. A micro preemie! I look over at that audience. They are emotionless statues. The mother looks exhausted. A vacancy in her eyes. I feel sorry for her because her journey shall not get easier with time. Her body shall heal from the delivery but she has a lot of work to do for the next few months. She'll be either pumping milk every 2 or 3 hours or she'll be awake worrying about the lack of milk. She shall be thinking about her baby and the next lab tests. She shall be burnt out and have days of depression. She does not anticipate the toll NICU shall take on her person-hood. Today she only thinks about her baby.

These are parts of the many monologues I hear. Like performances done in many reruns. Only the audiences changes. However the fear in the eyes remains the same.

The lights dim. It is curtain call. The loop continues.

Week 37

I am walking around the second-floor area where both the NICU and maternity sections are. I place my bag on the floor to look for milk at the bottom of it. My bag has my pump materials and all the things I shall need for an eleven-hour day. It is easy to lose something. While I dig around, a few people arrive to visit a new mother in her ward. Two of them stop to face the NICU. They start talking with pity in their eyes about the poor people who are stuck in there. There are sick babies in there, dying babies, and some are even in incubators. Wow, that sucks to be there. They went on as if it is a museum of torture, and they were slightly fascinated by it. I now have my milk out, raise myself and slowly make my way to the NICU. I do not look back as their sharp, shamed eyes pierce my back. All I hear is something like. 'oh my god,' I'm so sorry' Oh my god.' That must have been an awkward experience for them. But I just do not care. I do not look. For me, it is not new, and I have other things about which to worry. I am tempted to turn around with a smile to tell them that "it is okay; I did not hear anything" to lessen their embarrassment. Maybe I can just tell them that this place is full of heroes, tiny fighters who have achieved more in their lives then most adults. But I need to put this milk into the fridge and be there for his handling.

Newborn Feeding Schedule Milestone

Today his feeds are brought to every 3 hours, newborn schedule. It means that Elyot's tummy is big enough to hold this full load. It started with a slow drip of one millilitre, and daily they increased it while keeping it coming in slowly. This is something non micro preemie parents might take for granted, the timed meals.

The feeding tube causes his skin to be irritated. He hates it. I lost count of how many times he pulled it out. When he does this, it hurts him. The sticker holding it rips his skin.

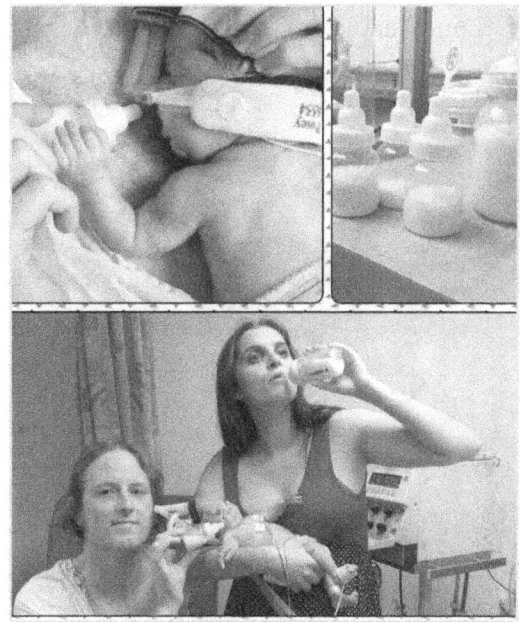

Week 38

Self Care

This is my last week of class. I am busy with finishing everything up. I had to battle my school to let me postpone my last semester. It is an internship semester and is physically impossible.

The crib makes a huge difference to my mood. I am permitted to decorate it as long as the objects are easy to sanitize plastic. For the first time after over three months here, I feel like we have a tiny apartment. It is so homey. I get to lean in, read to him books, and kiss his forehead while he sleeps. I try to draw again and work on my writing again. Somehow I am less sad now.

These weeks pass fast in these pages but in real life this is the slowest time. Urgency and worry no longer occupy me. I am just plain bored.

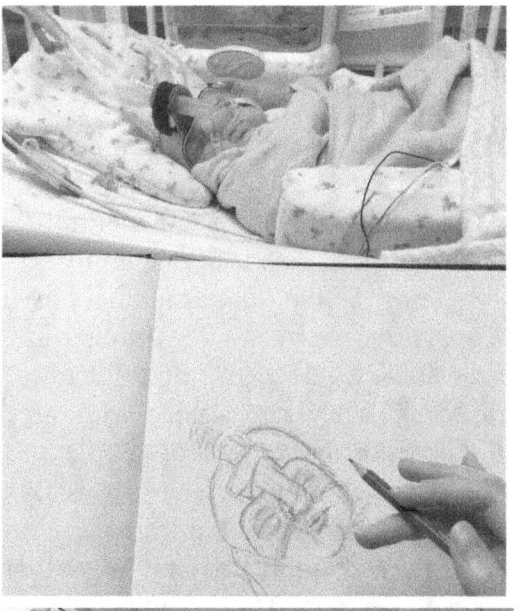

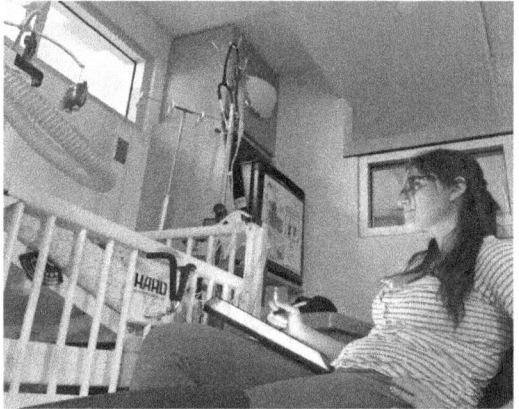

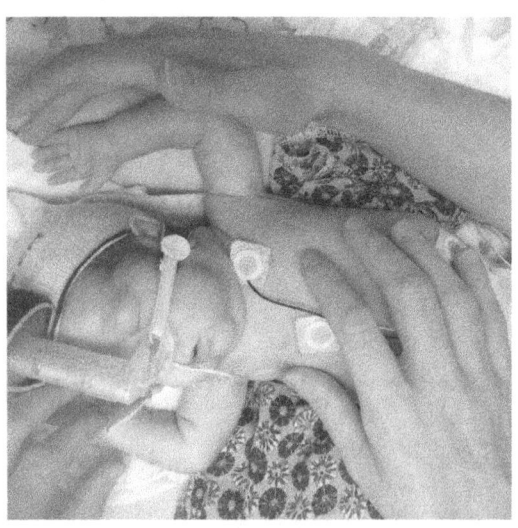

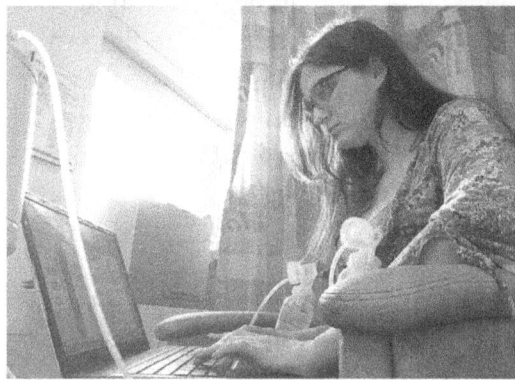

Not a Social Worker, a Demon

Malerie, my social worker, is at it again. She makes an appointment with me to have 'the talk'. In this talk, Malerie tells me that the staff here have been talking about me that I only do the bare minimum at the NICU. She explains that I only do one skin to skin, and he is now stronger and needs it twice a day. I have actually been waiting to do the two of them, but they said it is too soon and now she is here implying that I am lazy and neglecting him. I am already here for the whole day sitting next to him and holding him. I don't believe Malerie. Why could she not just tell me Elyot will benefit from more cuddle sessions? Why did she tell me that I am doing the minimum and pretend that the staff thinks I am neglectful?

She alone has made my suffering here beyond the words on this page. Now I look around, wondering if any of them called me lazy.

My hours now are about pumping 24/7, having a quick breakfast, one hour walk to the hospital, almost 11 hours with Elyot, then I do midnight pump, and the cycle continues. Burn-out isn't a strong enough word to explain how overwhelmed I am.

What do you label this feeling? It is almost a depression but not quite. I am exhausted, I am afraid, I am embarrassed. I am disappointed he is not coming home. I don't know what to hope for in Elyot's future.

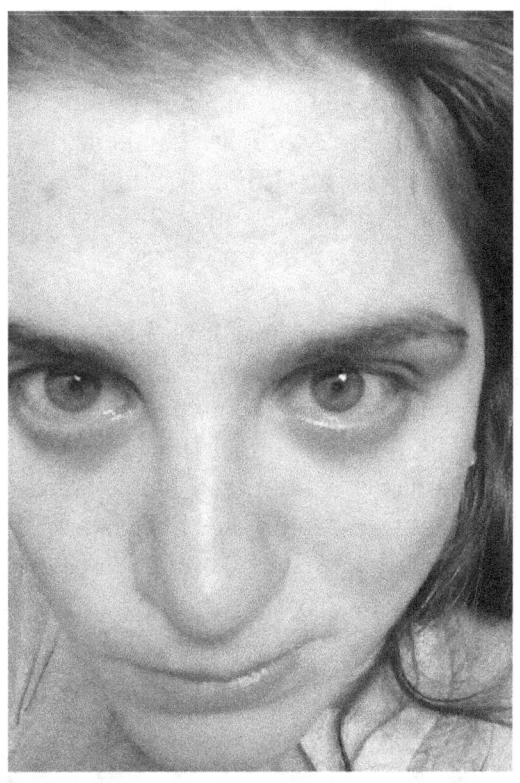

She tells me that my all is not enough.
She tells me to find water in a desert.
She tells me I am a bad mother.

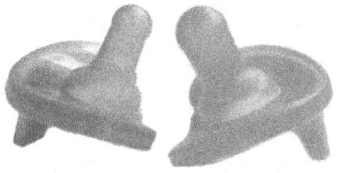

My body is returning to normal, so I begin to crave the return of my fitness. I think it means that the old Maria is finally coming back and realizing that she is a person. Since our NICU is now more relaxed, no one questions me if I sneak out to take a walk or close the curtains for some alone time or to try to do some exercises to try to return my splits. The nurses only come when they prepare his feeds. I am utterly alone with him, and I become accustomed to this solitude.

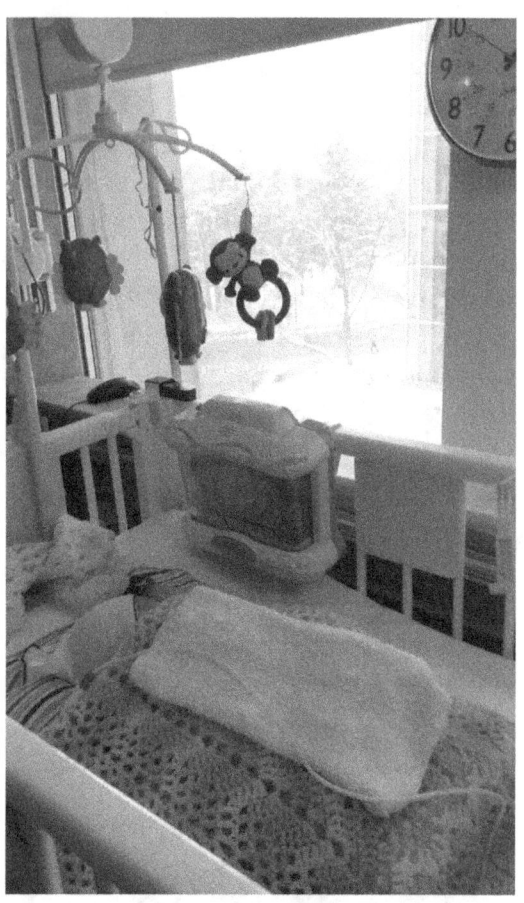

***

The nurses know how long I have been there and promised me that the minute a hub with a window gets freed, they shall give it to me. It is almost Christmas when it finally happens, and magical snow completes my vista. I am genuinely thankful and cheerful at this token of love.

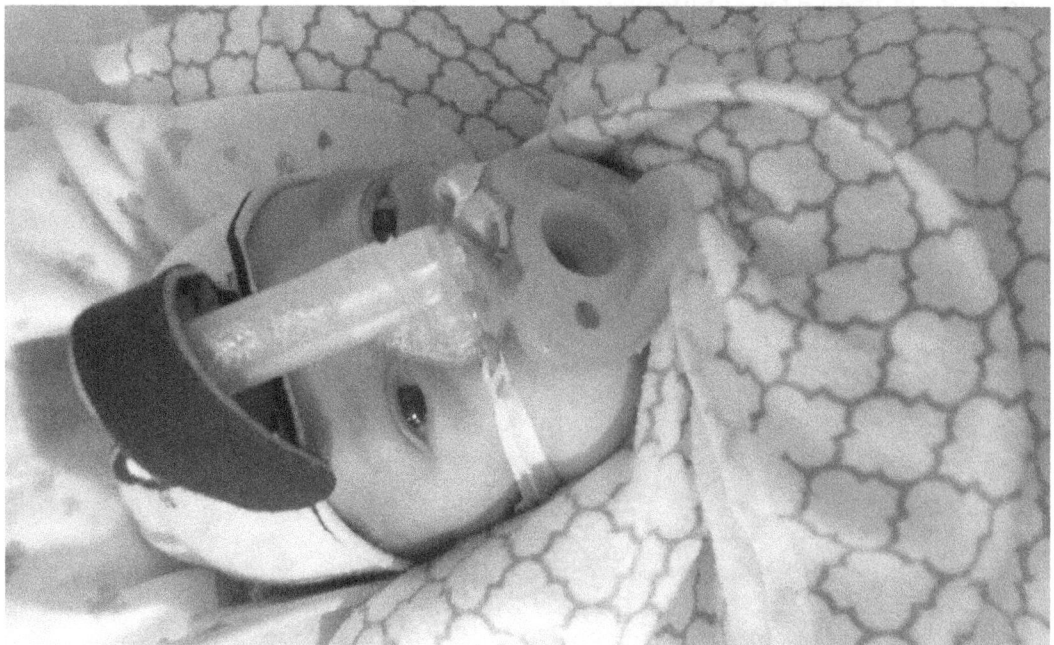

Week 39
No C PAP Milestone

It is the end of another uneventful week. We are closing into Elyot's due date. I am both cozy and have a slightly heavy heart as these holidays calendar milestones that are about to pass us by as if we do not exist. I walk into the hub; place my milk into the fridge; find a corner to put my backpack and what? I do a double-take. It is off! I see a face. His face. He is lying there looking around. Nose, lips, eyes, cheeks, everything. Where is the mask? I ask around a few times to confirm if this is a mistake. I scream so loudly with happiness that my neighbours join in my joy without knowing why I am excited. The lady next to me is new here and does not know about micro preemies. She is confused about why I am so excited. Her baby is here for a few day. I have no idea why. She hates it here. She does not understand why I'm jumping with joy. My happiness today is once in a life time! It is like nothing else. I would not trade places with that other mother who is very upset about being in the NICU for a few days.

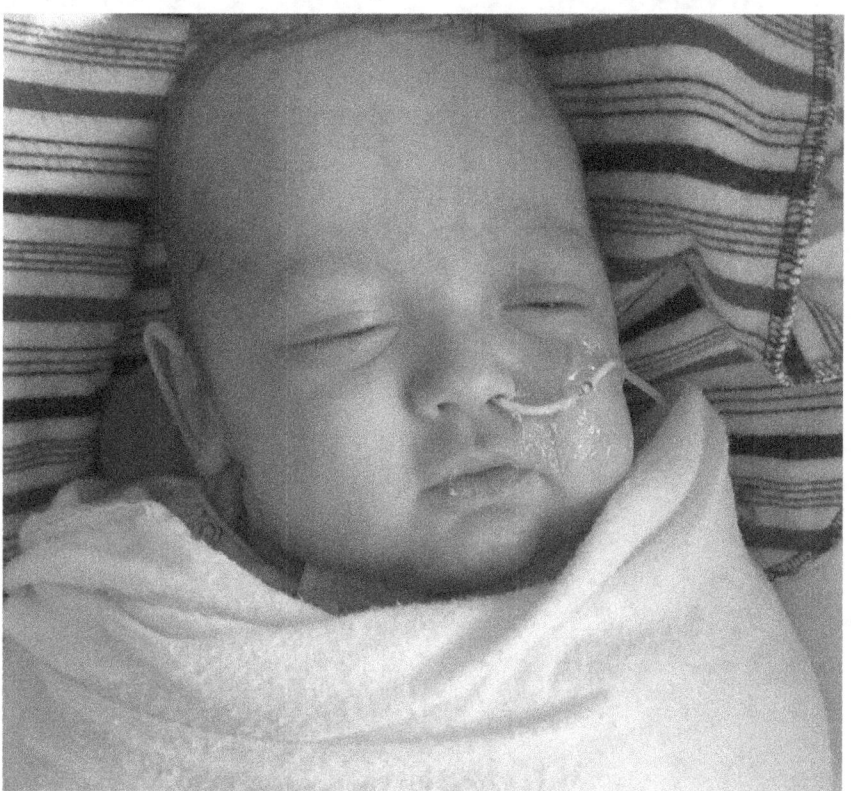

I come close to examine him and fill him with kisses. He has the typical egg-shaped head of which the internet warned. Premature babies long on the C PAP have a head like this from months of the tight hat that holds the mask. It will round off with time, but today it is an egg! A happy egg.

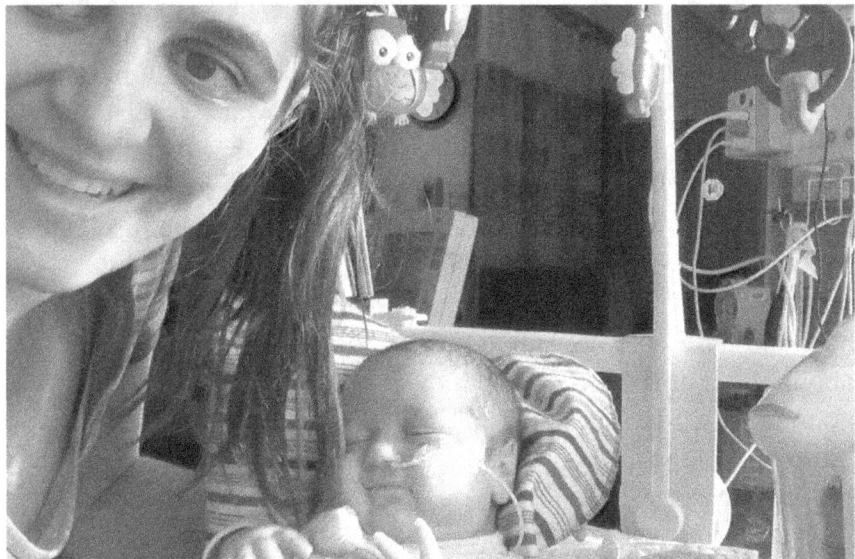

The nurse is glad that I arrived because he was taking up all her time, now that he has no mask on, he is bored and needs company. They give him a swing to entertain him, something impossible with a C PAP.

What does this mean that his mask is off? What am I allowed to hope for anything here where nothing is promised? Hope is not allowed here. They have seen to much. Hope is a risk. Just enjoy his face today.

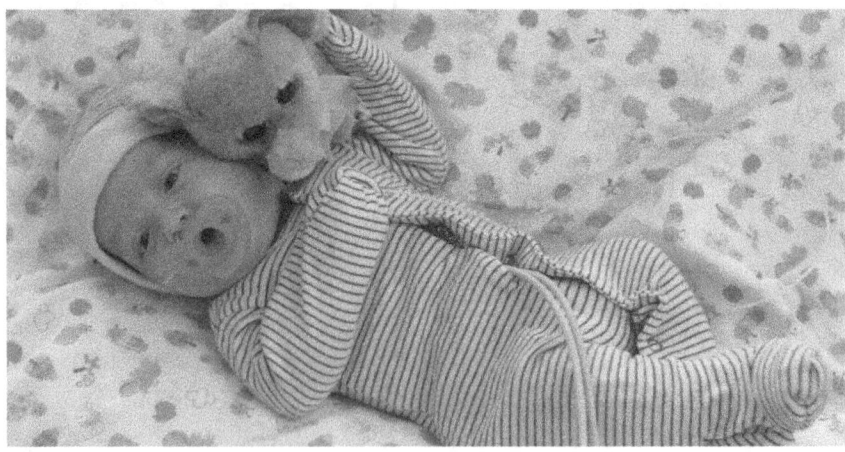

Up till this point, we have been told that his one-month low fluid made him more of a 24-week baby than a 25 week one and added to the severity of his lungs healing. He was supposed to go home with an oxygen tank and very likely a G tube into his belly because his lungs might prevent him from drinking milk. Today plans seem to have changed overnight. His mask hangs by his bedside as a superstitious thing. He needs to be able to breathe without the C PAP for five days before it is counted and before being allowed to be discharged to the less intense ward at Level 2. No one celebrates yet as they continue to continue to monitor his breathing. I am like a child with a new doll! So far, he does not need even that minimal support. He is free now so that I can dance with him across his hub. I close the curtains and prance around, enjoying him looking up at me. He is more attentive now, more social. He looks at me differently as if he only just noticed that I have a face.

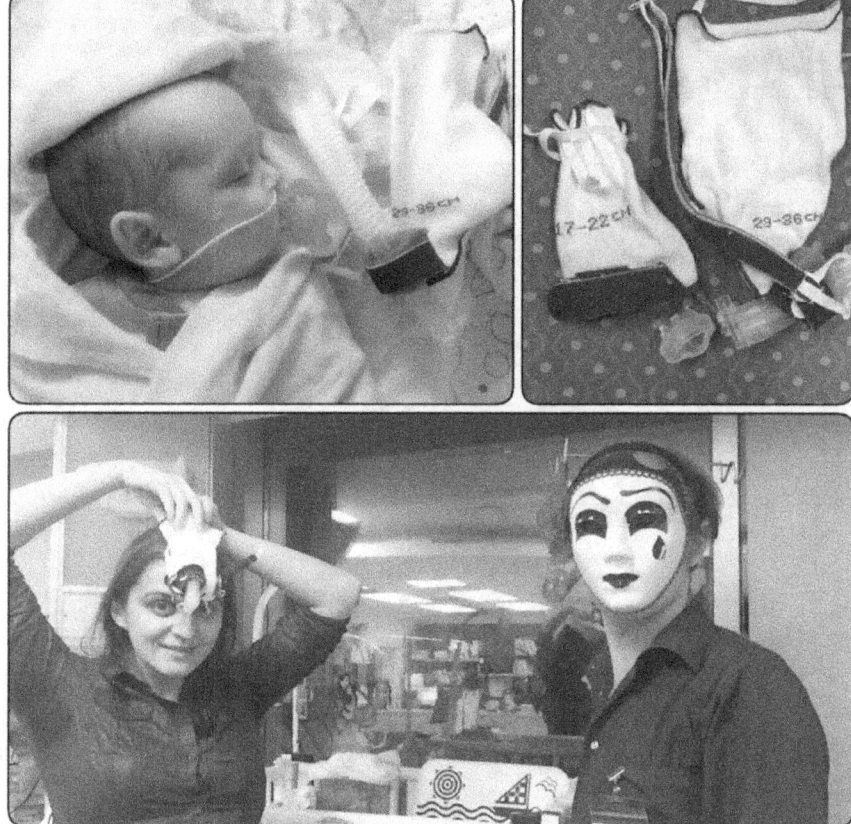

Week 40

Due Date

Today I give birth to him in a pool setting within a hospital with a midwife. Or maybe not. Maybe today, he is still NICU dependent but at least breathing on his own. All this is happening as if he understands that he is due to be born. He came off his breathing yesterday, and today is his due date. Nurses tell me to remain optimistic about the C PAP because it is his second day off it and did not desaturate [1] overnight. I am still in happy shock, but I try not to feel it in case if I lose it. They explain that once his scheduled days of air breathing are done, I can teach him to feed orally, and that journey might take months. I am no longer hoping to go home in January but understand that it might take longer.

They tell me to try breastfeeding immediately, and then if it does not work in the first month, then move to the bottle. The nurse sets up a meeting with a lactation consultant to start to work on it the minute the five days are up.

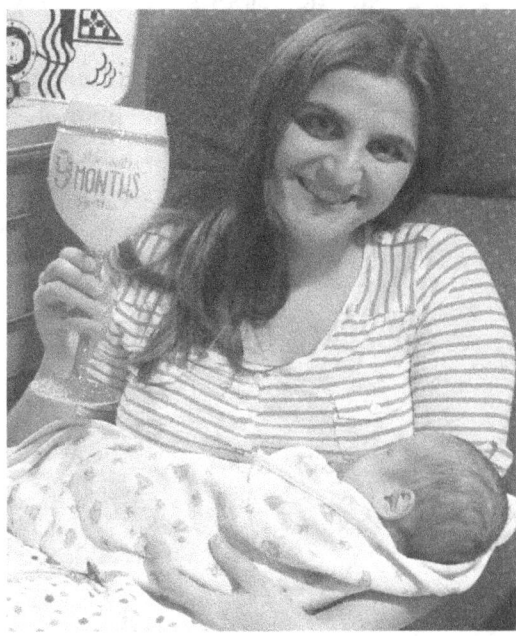

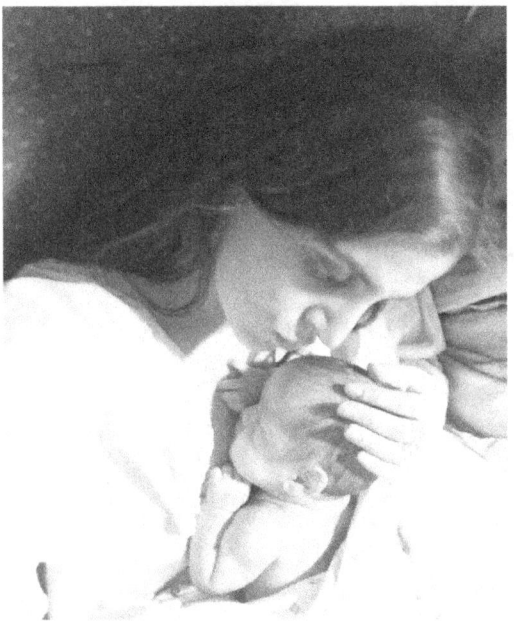

I have never experienced this togetherness. It is like we have been running to each other our whole lives, and finally, we get to lie cheek to cheek and rest. I still restrict myself from kisses, but I rub my face against his soft skin, I poke his chubby cheeks, and we stare into each others' eyes. Hi baby. Hi Elyot. I am pleased to meet you.

> His due date. Three and a half months after his legal date. He now has two birthdays.

---

1   desaturate - when oxygen is lower, most often at night.

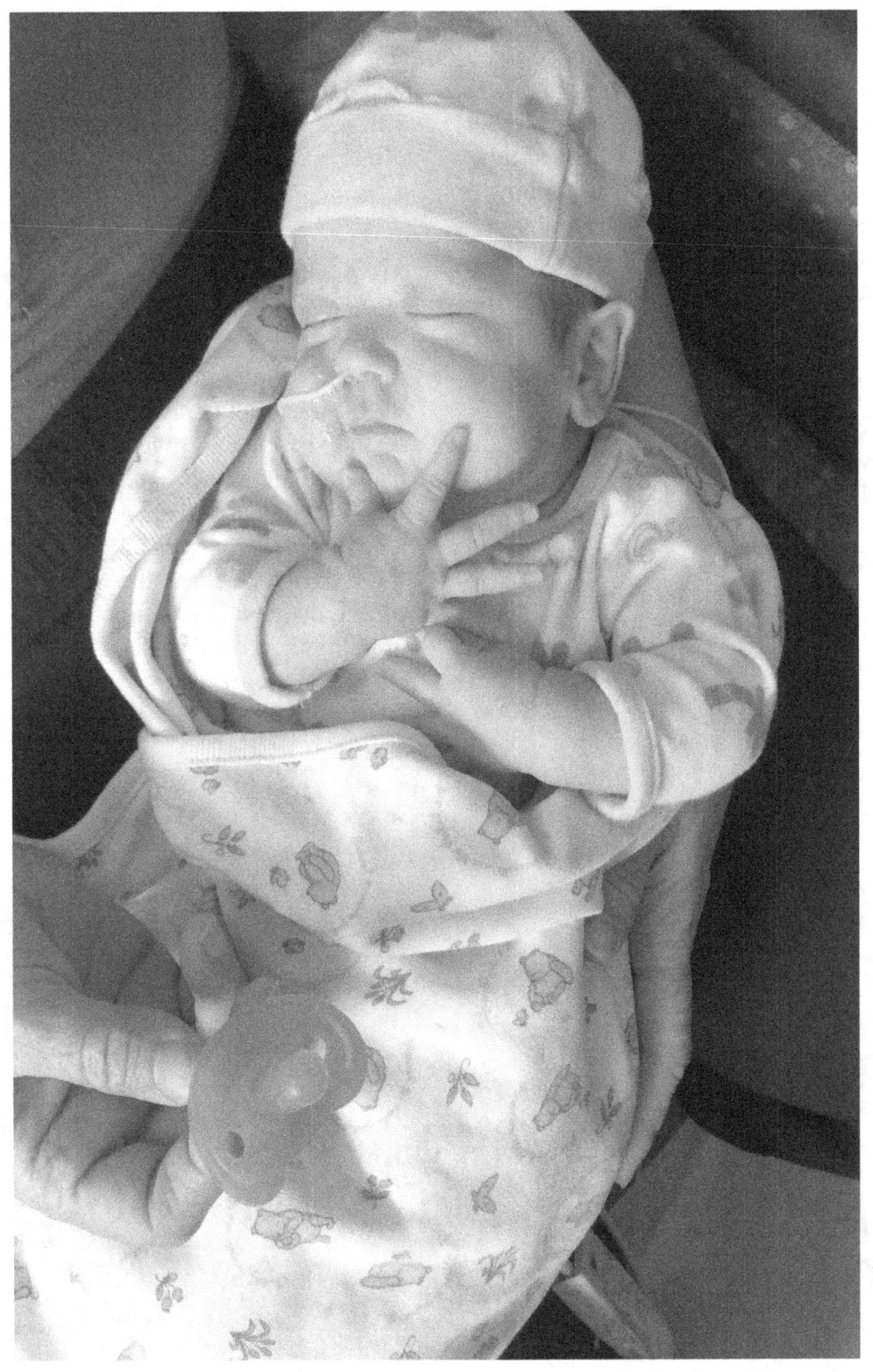

The next day my parents come from the United States. They planned to be here for his due date. Work did not give them time off earlier. My mother is in love. She arrives at the best time because he is looking up at her now. He was so passive and barely-there before. Now he wants to get to know who is holding him. He has a deep look at them as if he knows everything about you, and perhaps he does. If I can give Elyot a glimmer of love that I feel from my parents. How much I love you mama and papa but you live far away. Mama feels helpless being far away but a long story with immigration complications have separated us. Every year we try to reunite in either country. Now that Elyot is born I shall not visit to USA because of their pre-existing conditions and precarious healthcare.

My parents have to move here now. This is why I have so many photos included in this book. I share my life with my loved ones far away, every minute of my life.

My mother spends hours there. She has a major infection in her leg and it's not stopping her from coming to the hospital. I don't get to spend much time with her. She is my mama visiting and I wish we could hangout. But all her energy is for this little boy and to spend this time side by side with Maria. I celebrate these days for both of them. And the little fella gets tons of time with his grandmother, his babusia.

Sasha's perspective

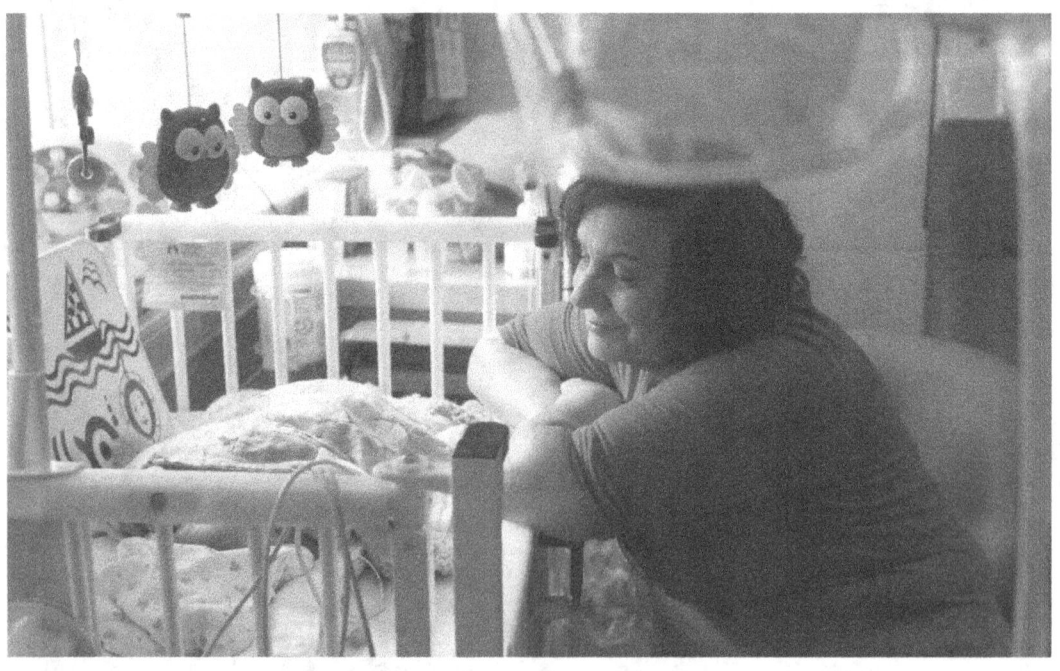

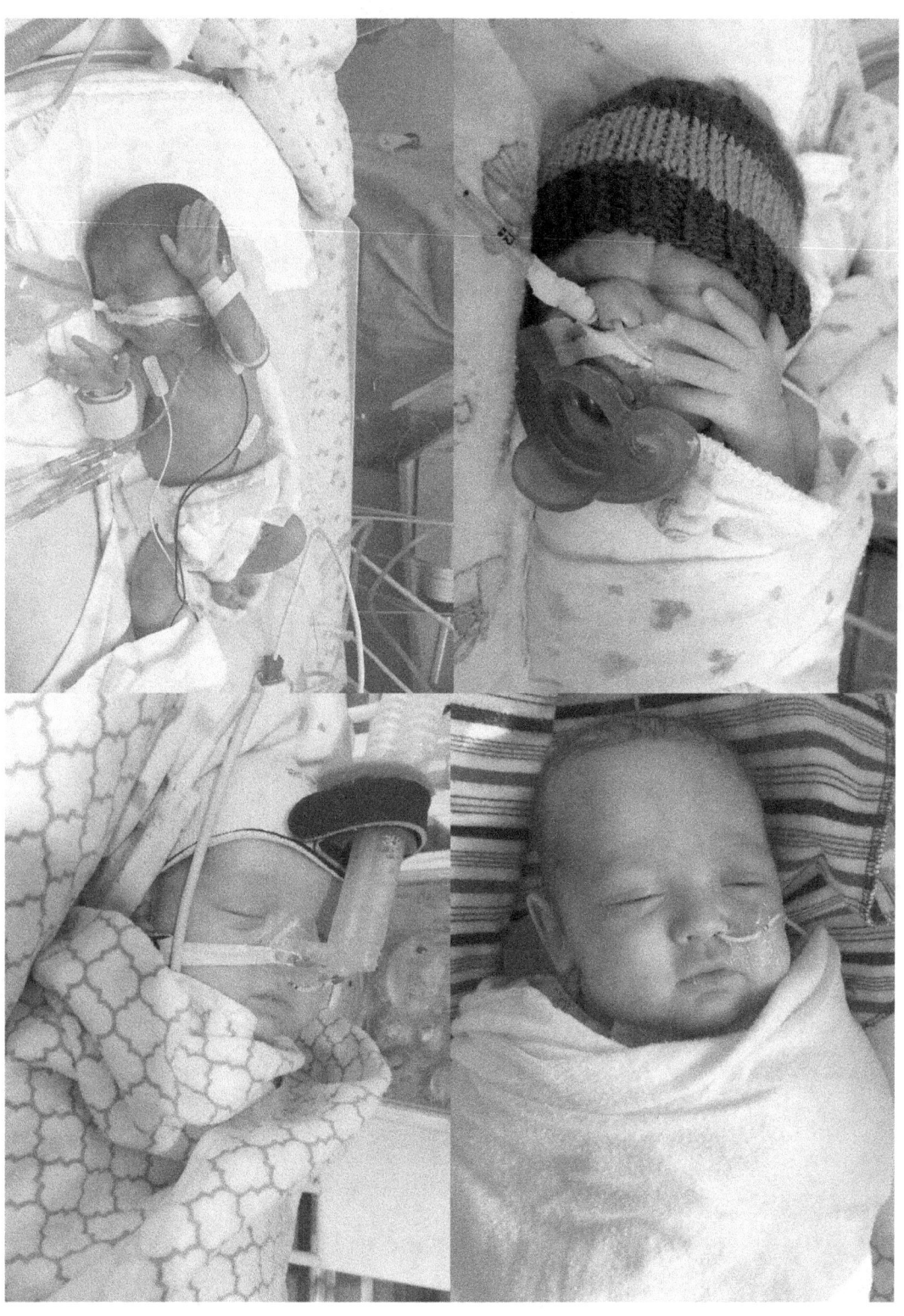

Chapter Four
The Last Battle

Level 2

Waking up to hear Elyot cry in the bassinet next to me as dawn peers in through the slit of the curtain, and the smell of coffee from the kitchen with the chatter of family somewhere echoes with the warmth of a home. We are home.

A dream. Yes, only a daydream. In reality, I wake up alone, pump, wait for mama, and we make the walk over the crunchy frosty early morning snow to spend the day with Elyot. Mama will leave halfway to be home with my pregnant sister, and I shall remain here till night.

After Elyot proves to be strong enough without breathing support for five days, they move us to another section of the NICU called Level 2. It is a place for less sick, less premature babies who need short-term support. It is very a clinical and bright, giant space with everyone almost next to each other. No curtains for privacy, no personal fridges.

There is no ambience of a mini apartment, but rather more like a busy supermarket. An assembly line that needs to get these babies out as soon as possible.

Hardly anyone is in an isolette here, so you hear crying babies from the cribs all day long. Elyot seems to be the only one with no cry. His lungs are weak, so his cry is only audible up close. You also see everyone's monitors, and their oxygen is at 100 percent. Ours is 98 in the day and goes to 96 at night. I get angry and envious about the 100 percent. The primary issue babies suffer here is being born a tad too small, so the nurses are working on fattening them up and make sure they can eat before they leave. Most stay a few days. Those born around 34 weeks are treated for jaundice and go to other less intensive hospitals. Level 2 is short-term. It is not a journey; it is a crib that needs to be emptied for the next patient as soon as possible.

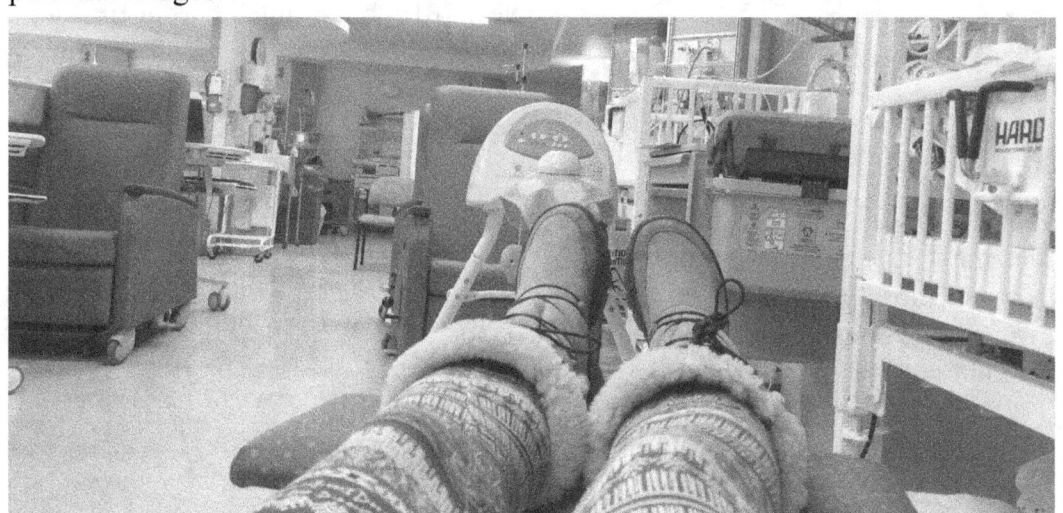

They see what looks like blood in Elyot's stool, so they have to put us into isolation. It means that you need to wear gloves and a robe every time you are close to your baby. It is a tedious extra thing to do, but one becomes used to it very quickly. They do not want Elyot's whatever's spreading to others.

Mama makes it fun. We joke around a lot wearing this protective gear. It reminds us of old Soviet movies we'd watch about lab experiments. We laugh a lot. Why not laugh? He is breathing independently, and my whole family is with me, even if not at the NICU but at least at home, waiting for me with a warm meal and a hug.

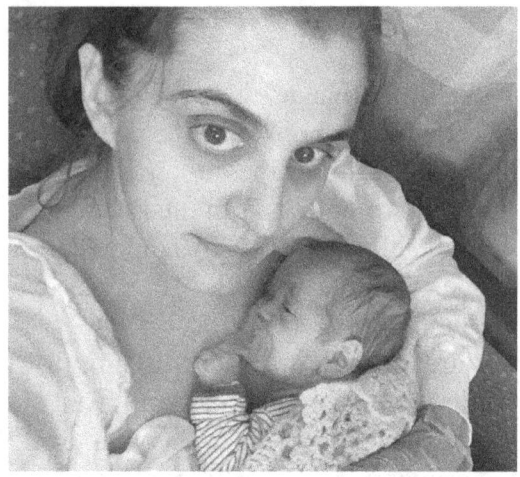

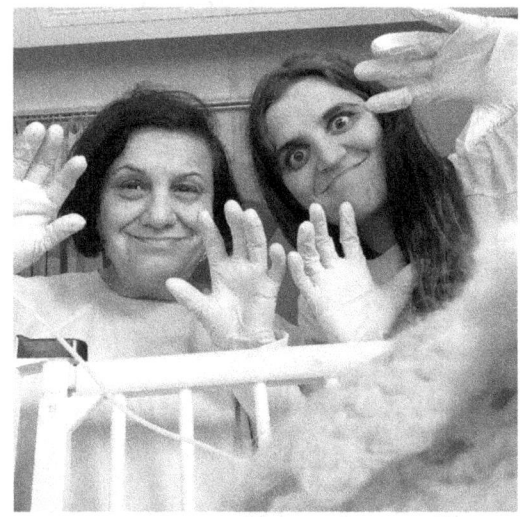

We have to wait until Elyot's tests return negative before we can be freed from isolation. I remind them about my lactation consultant. I am eager to begin breastfeeding.

It is the year 2020 of the infamous Covid 19 virus as I write this book. Another story altogether, but now as I look back at this time in 2016, little did we know that this isolation is nothing compared to what is to come in the future. I am pregnant again, resting; this is why I have time to write this book. I shall update you at the end on how this second pregnancy works out since I do not know yet. But what I can tell you now is that I do not want to be part of a hospital stay during a deadly pandemic. No matter how bad the year 2016, it is a much harder time for anyone in 2020. In 2016 both parents are allowed in or two visitors as long as one is the parent. Many NICUs in 2020 only allow one parent in. You have to do strict screenings to come inside and always wear a mask. No extra items are permitted in 2020, unlike in 2016, where I bring in my books and sketch pads. Also, our greatest threat back then is the RSV virus, not RSV and Covid 19.   Covid 19

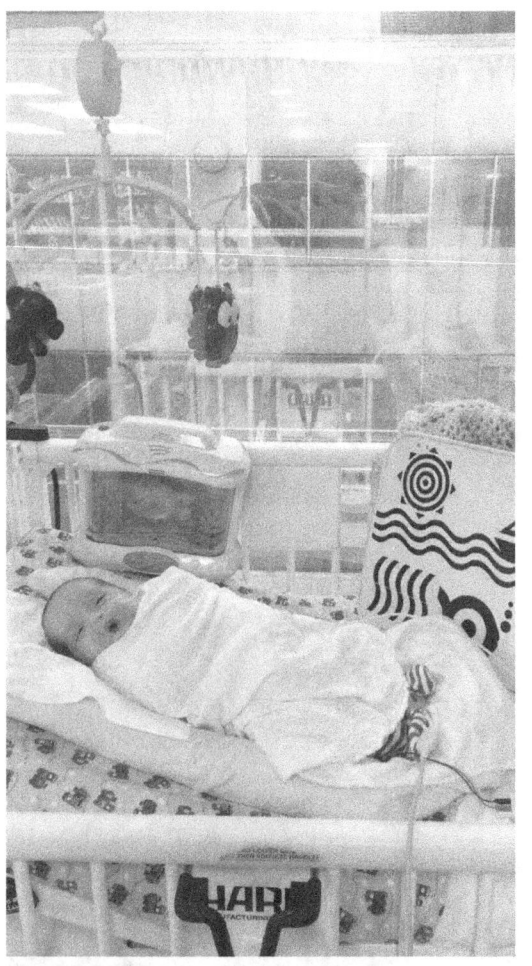

Most micro preemies do not latch and become bottle babies. I do not expect anything. My main goal is to last two years with breast milk because his immune system will be low for a while.. Statistics show that pumping does not last long, usually not lasting more than six months, and I badly want to last long. So far, I have been pumping for four months, and I am close to that statistic where many parents begin to lose their milk.

We are about two weeks after his due date, and these cute outfits are getting wasted. I try to make him wear as many of them as possible to at least get some use out of them. He is big for his size and already outgrowing newborn clothes. That answer to the question of what size he shall be when he is be at his due date is that he is almost too big to be a newborn; by next week, we start to bring in 0 -3 size in which is the next size from newborn. And there, we thought he would be too small.

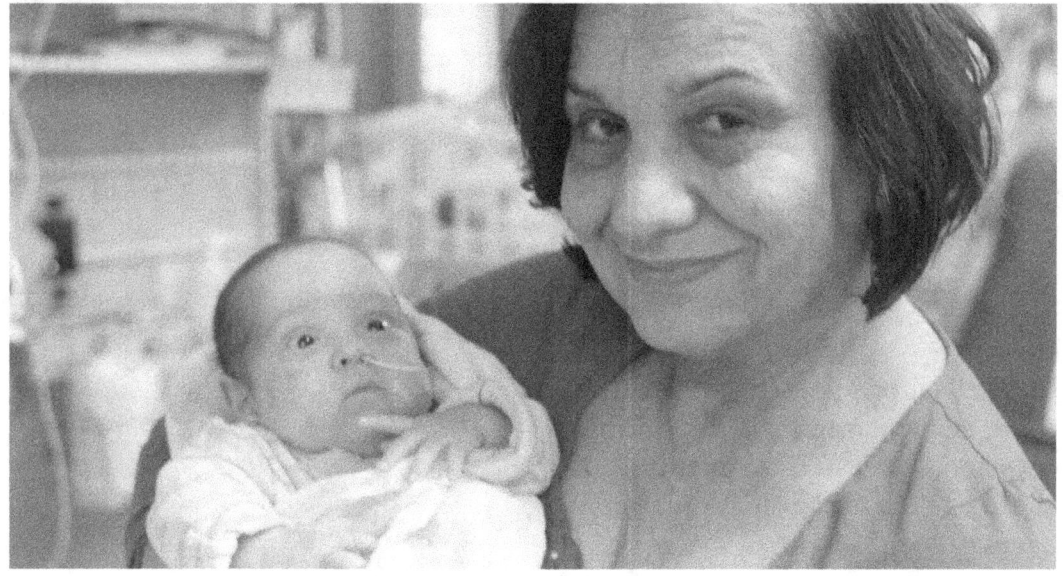

Christmas and New Years

We do not do anything celebratory for Christmas because what is the point? I am still a guest resident at my sister's house. Geoff still lives in Yorkton. Christmas is a set of sterile white lights in a cold spaceship. Milestone photos and dressing up are no longer fun. I am just doing this because I started it. We do have a few family and friends visiting one by one to see Elyot. However, that proves exhausting because you repeat your script to each person about how he is doing, what all the equipment is, and reassure them that I am doing well. Geoff and I meet them in the cafeteria and take turns bringing them because Level 2 has the same two-person rule. In 2020 you will not have an open cafeteria and friends visiting.

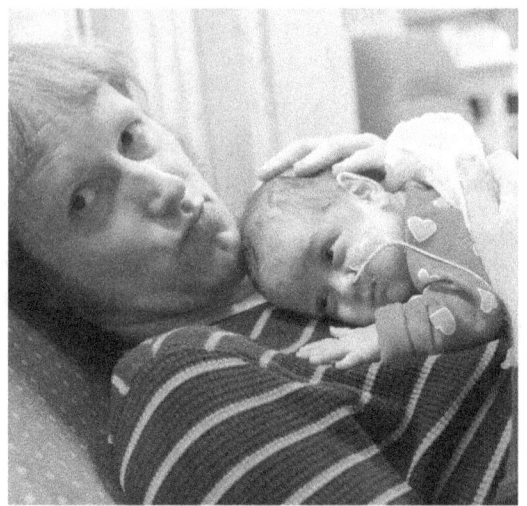

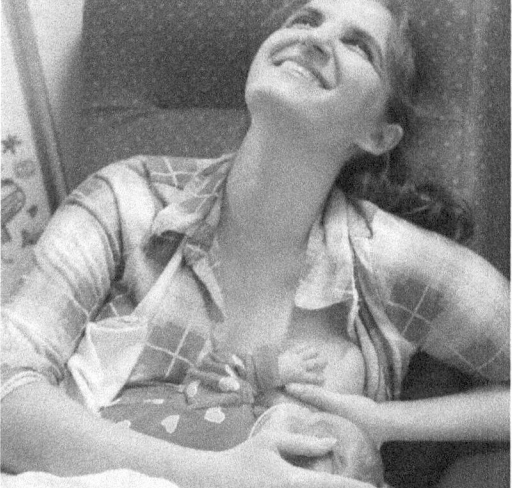

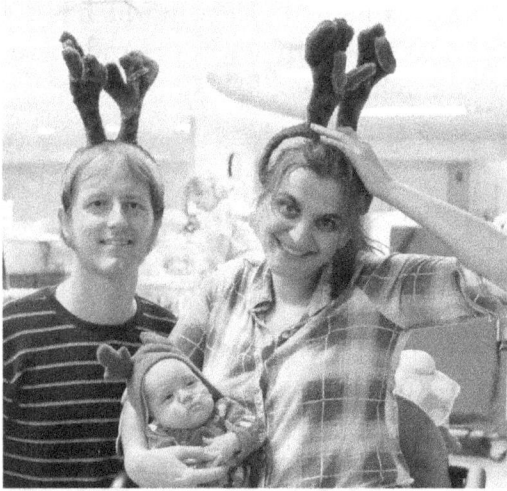

The staff surprise us with gifts and cards, and volunteers make food. It does boost morale. But it is still lonely. However cold this place is, it is our home today.

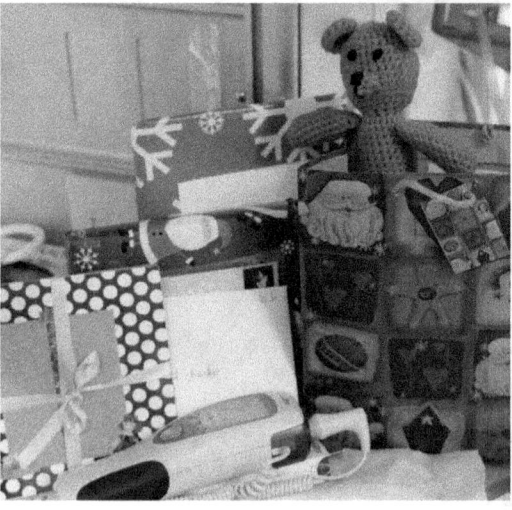

My parents leave the next day after Christmas because they have to work. It all goes downhill once they depart. The low-frequency breathing nasal prongs surprise us today. He showed himself off to his loving visitors but now he wants to rest. This breaks my heart.

He hates the tube. His mood is instantly down. The curious creature he used to be is now no longer. Also, he cannot breastfeed until this tube is gone; we are forced to put it on a break. I have been working on breastfeeding on my own up to this point but I have no idea what I am doing. No lactation consultant came to me. I try to not lose time. But now the tube is forcing us to stop anyways.

New Years is not a celebration. We visit him as usual and go home. Geoff goes to sleep; I continue pumping through the night. It is extra quiet there during the eve of New Year. No babies are crying. It feels like maybe there are fewer people here during this time.

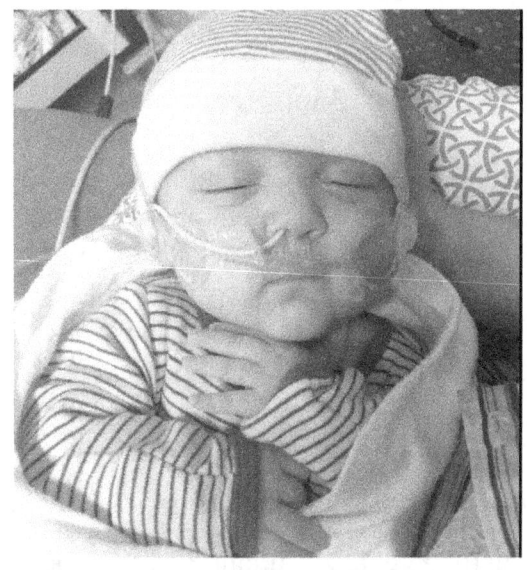

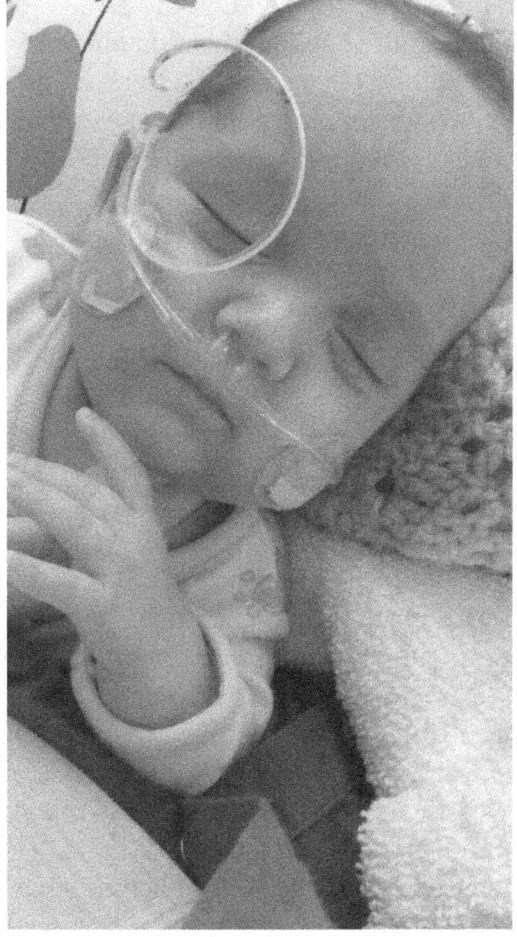

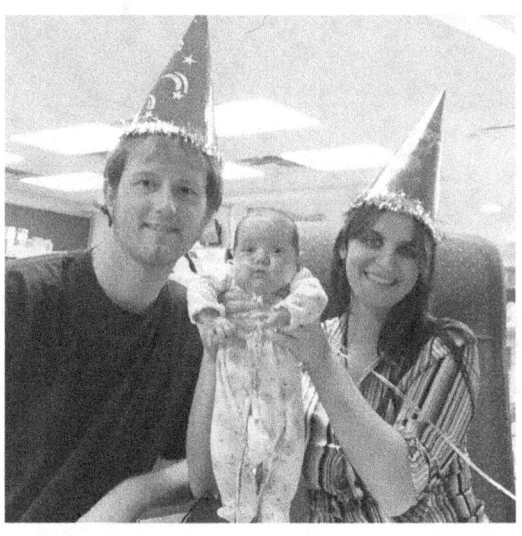

4 Months

Bunk Room

It has been a whole month now since Elyot came off his breathing devices. We were supposed to get started on breastfeeding right away. The holidays made most of the staff be away, then when they returned there were communication issues. I go up to the front desk of Level 2 unit to try again because I have seen others with help. It is a big jumble of confusion, but eventually, I get a consultant. Level 2 does not have the organization of Level 3. There is little communication among the staff here. I am thrilled to be here, but also beginning to get upset because we are going home a month later now.

My consultant specializes in micro-preemie troubles and is very helpful right away. She says Elyot's mouth pallet is deeper than their babies because of the tube in his mouth while he was growing, so he shall have to work harder to learn to latch or drink. This is to add to our month lost. I no longer dream of Valentine's Day to be home. But it no longer matters. I am here now for as long as it takes for Elyot. Once I stop dreaming of home, I can put all my efforts into him. She sets up a schedule and advocates for me to get a bunk room next to the NICU. I would live in it and work on breastfeeding every three hours around the clock. I'm so happy. I ask my family to bring me stuff, pyjamas and food for the night. The NICU arranges to phone me when Elyot wakes up at night. Practical questions arise. How shall I juggle nightly pumps with Elyot every three hours? Do I pump first or after?

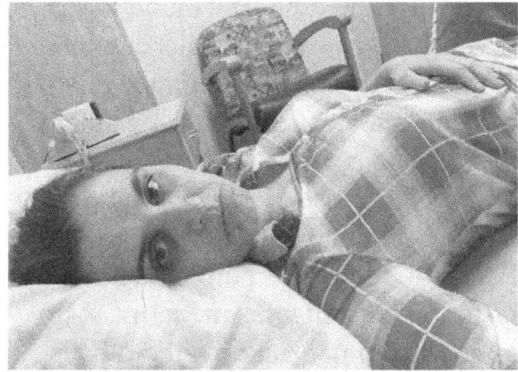

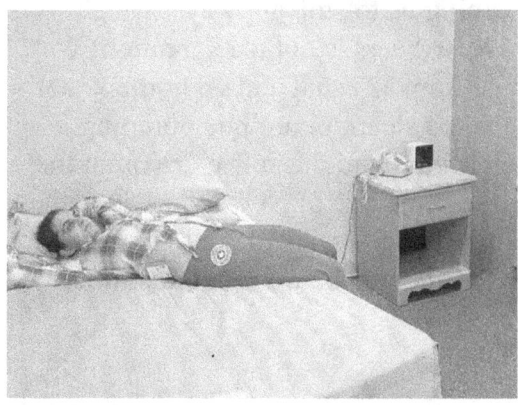

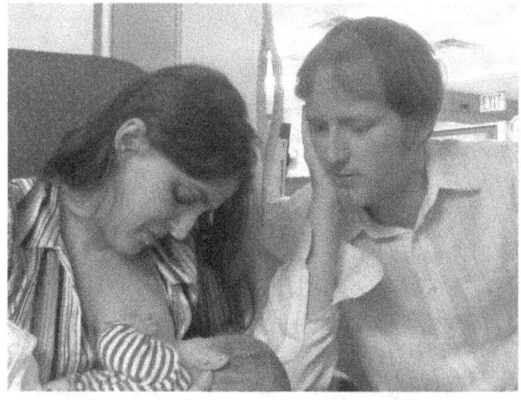

If you didn't do the bunk train, you don't know suffering. If the NICU is a jail, this is the isolation chamber. It is musty, no windows and slightly chilly. Yet this box is my heaven, my new excitement for what the future shall bring.

My first cycle is a nightmare. Elyot cries his most desperate cry that I have ever seen. A scream so strong that his lungs cannot produce a sound. He is hungry, but the milk does not come fast enough for him. I cry in return.

When Geoff took this photo of Maria, it was her happiest moment since the whole ordeal started. She left my house with a skip in her step. I have not seen her like this for a long time. She had a plan. It was written out in her calendar at home. We had a big conference all with all the family as she announced her next two weeks. Unfortunately this does not last.
This is her first and her last night of pure joy until it goes downhill.

Sasha's perspective

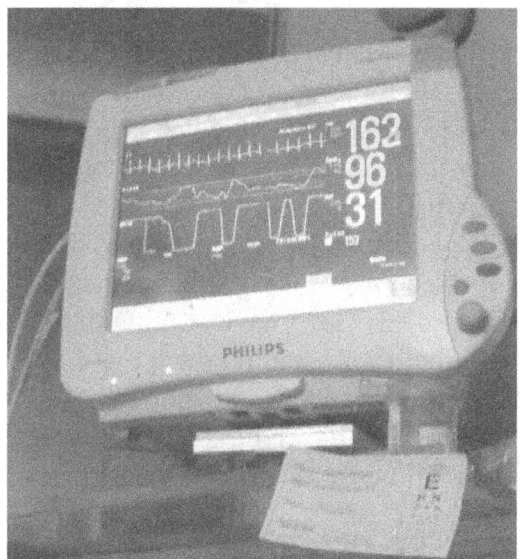

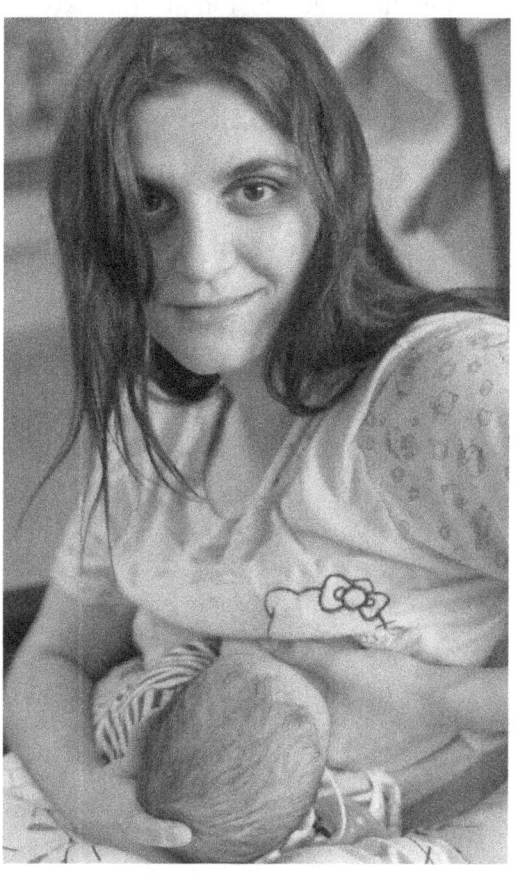

How it is done. You weigh him. You try to feed him – both cry. You weigh him again. Every gram gained is a millilitre of milk consumed. You return him to his crib, start up his feed that you have been warming the whole time. Pump, sanitize the pumps, label the milk – then you go to bed with one last look at Elyot as you walk by. In bed, you have a small cry but also hope.

Mother Vs Malerie

The first night of bunk room in the bag. Many more to go. I now understand how hard this will be, but I have never been so motivated for something. I did not get much sleep because of this schedule. Elyot slept through the three am, so we missed that one. I have mixed feelings about it. On the one hand, it gave me a break, but also it was a session we missed, and every session seems to be better than the previous one. Otherwise, we both survived crying every three hours until a somewhat nice session at nine. Not bad for a result first thing in the morning and something to brag about to family when they call. Now I hope to get some milk into Elyot for 12; then, I shall pump and have a nap to catch up on sleep lost. My sister can sit with him while I take these naps so that he is never alone. Great plan, I am excited. I arrive at my routine.

Pump ready to go for later, milk syringe warming up for Elyot, and the breastfeeding pillow prepared to go. The doctor on duty approaches and tells me they are moving me to Northville later today, to start packing. I am confused. I tell them that it must be a mistake because I just started a bunk room thing with breastfeeding. They respond that all the paperwork was done because the social worker said I want to move on. My hands are shaking as I tighten them against the crib, and tears are flowing with free will. Elyot is waking up hoping for a meal. I have so many questions, and I wish I had family to help as I choke on everything that I am saying.

Firstly, doctor, I did not consent to leave because I have a minimum of a two-week plan to breastfeed. Secondly, why Northville? I have nothing to do with that city. I remind them that I live here in Hamtown for a while after our discharge while Elyot is high risk. This is my home for now.

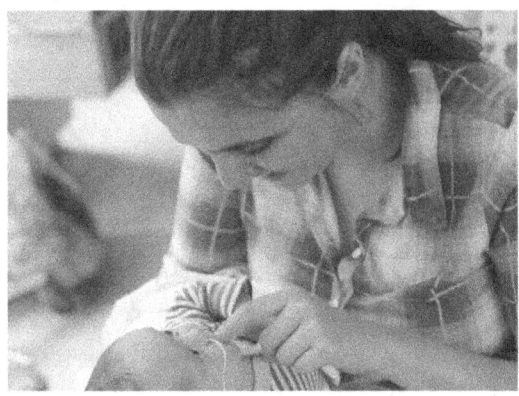

Now I am late for the noon feed!

Northville is too far for me. It is a lengthy bus ride and I would lose all my family supports. Even if she tried to get me back into a Yorkville hospital that originally rejected me, that one is at least close to my Yorkton home. She also refuses the closer Hamtown Level 2 hospital. Both those options have family who is close. Why all the way in Northville?

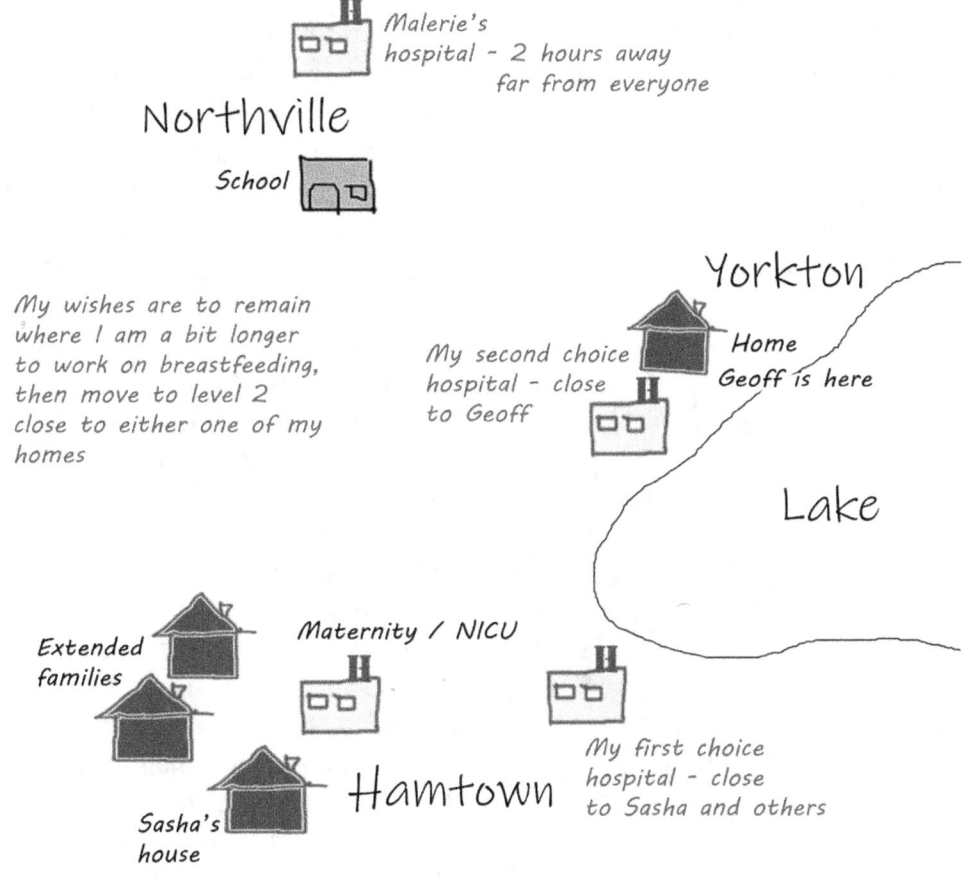

She went behind my back and lied that I want to leave. Why would I arrange the bunk room? My lactation consultant is thinking ahead. My impression is I am here to stay till we decide if breastfeeding will work out. I have a month to do this as they recommended. Those other hospitals do not have bunk rooms, so they cannot continue these lessons. I wonder if Malerie told them to send Elyot to Northville because that is where my school was. An act of petty revenge for something she hated me doing this whole time. I always tried to get replacement caregivers for Elyot on those days, and she is the one who refused it, so I lied and used my sister on those hard days when Elyot got his shots and needed to be held. She could have chosen Yorkton or, even better, Hamtown; why Northville?

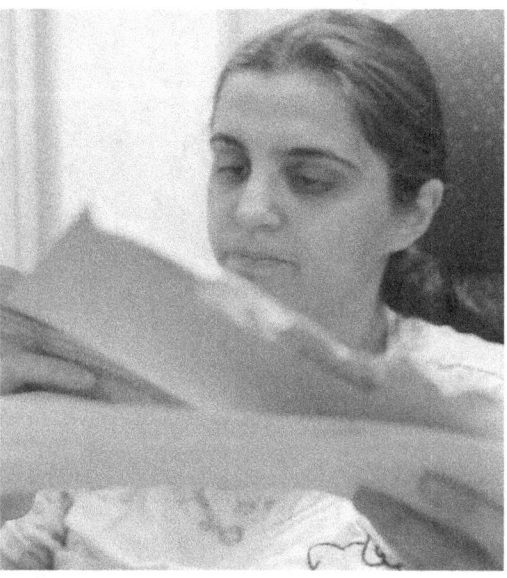

Up to this point, I thought she was just a bad social worker; now I see she is petty and evil.

Sorting through mail to prove where I live. The doctor walks away, and another person comes and tells me I am leaving today. They have a clear script prepared. I have seen it with other parents who did not want to go. My problem is that they promised me breastfeeding; even their inspirational posters in the pump room lectured me about how important it is. I am now five months pumping and do not know how long the milk will last like this. Elyot will be sickly in his first years of life. I am trying to get him stronger. Much to my embarrassment, the whole Level 2 room is now looking at me. Many of them already pity me with my back story, and I have been trying so hard to look positive in front of them. Also, the doctors are digging into my feeding session already. I have never seen these doctors before. I have no idea who we are. They are not talking to Maria with her Elyot but rather to a chart full of numbers no longer needed in this Level 2.

After the hassle of this morning, finally, Malerie appears, and I explain that there was a mistake. Instead of trying to understand, she repeats her talking points about how I actually live in Yorkton and that it is a lie if I stay in Hamtown. Feeling hopeless, I ask if there any hospitals in Yorkton at least.

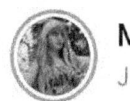

Maria Zak
January 6, 2017

So we just came up with a plan to teach Elyot to learn to feed orally. I moved into their little room to be here for every feed. Suddenly they want to discharge me to another community hospital that has no feeding plans or rooms to stay in. No consideration that he can't even eat yet. So I made such a huge fuss. Cried at the top of my lungs and threatened to chain myself to the crib. Don't know what will happen to us in the next few days but McMaster Hospital has no heart. I'm not going quietly. And we're also documenting all this and it's going into the documentary for sure! Thanks Mac for giving this film the perfect conflict moment it needs.

She insists that she wants me to go to Northville. Why there? No one lives there? Why there? Unsure what is left to do because everything I say to Malerie, she changes into her narrative, and uncertain if the NICU heads are getting my actual message, I write it out in a note. It is a desperate last chess move of a mother fighting for the future health of her son who has a severe lung problem. While they disappear to discuss me, I struggle through this feeding session. Elyot does fine with his tiny gulps until he falls asleep. I put his passed-out little body in the crib, swaddle him and start to pump at his bedside, afraid to leave him. While pumping, I complete my note. They have threatened us, Elyot. I am here for you. There is nothing I will not do for you. You are my strength. Now sleep, little one, and we shall try again at three.

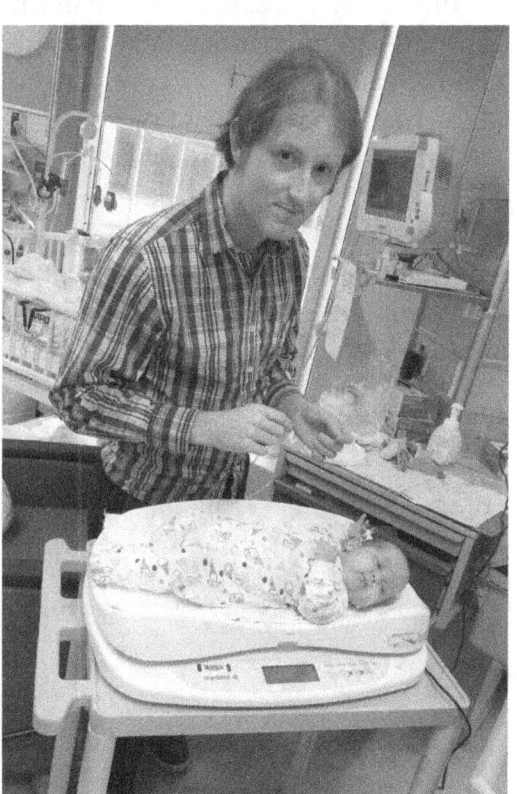

You weigh him, then feed him, then reweigh him. That is how you know how much he drank.

The letter seems to have done it. They leave me alone for another day. But the innocence is gone. Malerie will be coming after me so much that I beg nurses not to tell her where I am. She always finds me.

The nurses do not believe me when I try to tell them what is happening. I ask for advice, but they say nothing. Either they know her and are afraid, or they do not believe me, in which case she told them something about me like last time when she said everyone in the previous ward thinks I am lazy. A mere 24 hours pass, and she is here again telling me they need the bunk room.

She tries to change her approach now. Instead of kicking me out to free a room, she now thinks she is helping me with ideas. She suggests I go home, sleep there, have a bath and a good meal, and return here with a taxi for each night feed.

I explain that I have no money for a taxi. I either need a bed elsewhere in the building or a bunk room. She says there is no bed anywhere and that no matter what my bunk room is finished. There is nowhere in the hospital that I can sleep.

When she is gone, and doctors come to ask me about my plans, I tell them with tears more enormous than Jupiter thunderstorms that I am going nowhere. I am going to chain myself to this crib, and I am not leaving. They treat the bunk room as a luxury as if we really want to be there because it is fun. There is neither empathy nor understanding of how hard it is for us. It would have been easier to give up and take what they offered but...him.

I AM GOING TO CHAIN MYSELF TO HIS CRIB

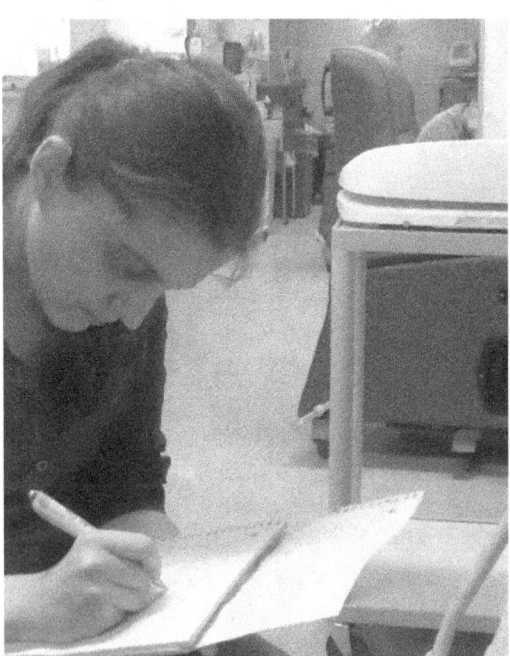

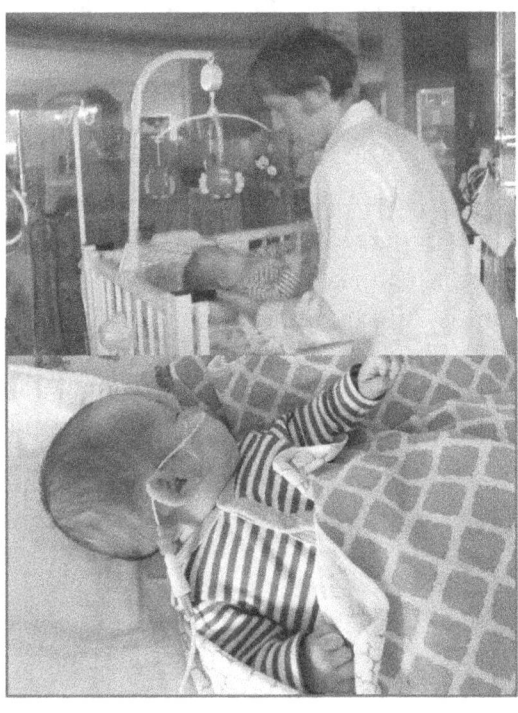

8 January 2016

Re: Discharge Plans

I, Maria [REDACTED] reside in Ham[REDACTED] and have lived here for 8 months already and plan to live here for some time after discharge from hospital. Since [REDACTED] Hospital is the closest to me, it makes sense to discharge us to [REDACTED]'s Hospital in Ham[REDACTED]. There has been some confusion about the discharge location so I am clarifying it here and it shall not change at any point. I live here, I have all of my support here and shall get support right after a complete discharge.

Also I ask for some advocacy for us when we are discharged to [REDACTED] in Ham[REDACTED] to have a continuity of care and support about our attempts to breastfeed. I want to maintain my milk supply for 2 years to give my boy the best in his quality of life and I believe it is worth it to attempt breastfeeding. I live off a single income and I have no car so my options are limited. Please can we continue our work on breastfeeding at [REDACTED]'s in Ham[REDACTED], but only with your help, can that be possible.

Thank you for everything you have done for us! We love you and shall be grateful for the rest of our lives.

Maria
[REDACTED]

Maria Zak ▶ Elyot The Inspiration
13 January 2017

So I just talked to another mom of a 25 week baby. She also has ␣lerie as a social worker. She hates ␣lerie too. It's not just me! Also they are treated differently because of their long term problems too. It's definitely a pattern to prioritize people who are quicker than those who have long term needs. Not just us.

We weigh him, feed him, reweigh him and scream with joy because it is working. Elyot works hard, and we are getting fast results. He gets tired at every session and turns into a floppy doll but gets more milk in each time. Geoff tries to be here as often as he can at night time to help me. You have up till now witnessed my struggle, but here is the daddy doing his best to help with morale, weight taking and pump washing. It is a whole family event. We are all working hard to achieve this. Plus, Elyot is reaching his 100 SAT score for the first time in a long time because though he gets tired, he loves every minute of this.

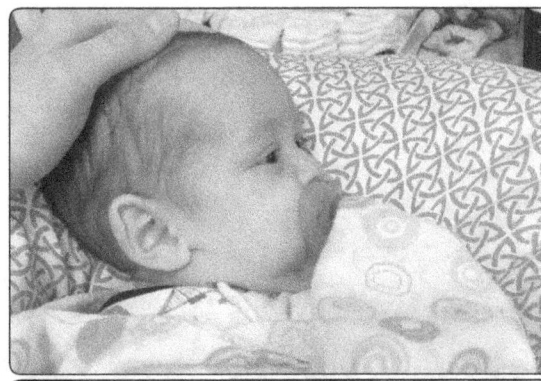

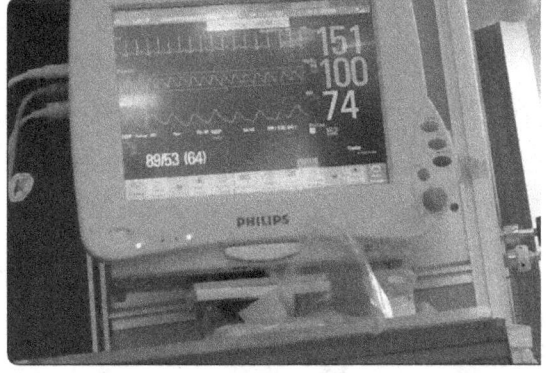

 Maria Zak ▶ Elyot The Inspiration
15 January 2017

We fired our social worker! Maybe too soon because Elyot made such progress in the last 24 hours that I don't get to gloat in her face. She didn't believe me that it'll work with feeds.

If I bump into her I'll tell her that we replaced her because we needed

The Luxury

If anyone did any breastfeeding or pumping, they might know about inflammation. While balancing Elyot and then working on pumping, it confuses the body, and the milk glands turn to rocks. I start getting sick a couple of days into this schedule. I think that I am catching a cold; I do not know that this is inflammation from inconsistent nursing. I am freezing. I put on every layer of clothing that I can find. I sneak in a heater and sit next to it. Nothing helps to warm me up.

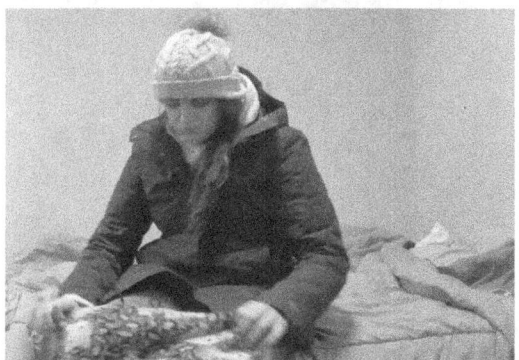

To add to this, I have stress from fear of being kicked out of the bunk room staring at me daily. I start to lose milk. I am in panic mode. Twice when I attended night feeds, I almost fainted. I skip one three am feed I because I am too weak to get out of bed. That morning, I get the message that I shall lose the bunk if I don't show up. I can see the pattern now. They do not want me there. They think because Elyot is a micro-preemie, he won't reach his targets, so it is a waste of a room.

Many more mothers join Level 2. Their babies are healthy. They just need to work on breastfeeding. I know they want to kick me out to give them the room. It is so much pressure that I start risking fainting, but I make sure to show up to every feed. No one explains the pumping process. No one explains that a person feels flu symptoms from inflammation. I am desperate to get better so that I have the energy to continue the bunk train. Any mistake will get me kicked out. I stop crying because I have no more energy. It is that same autopilot mode I had when Elyot was first born. You ignore your sickness, crusty red eyes and blistered nipples and do what you need to do.

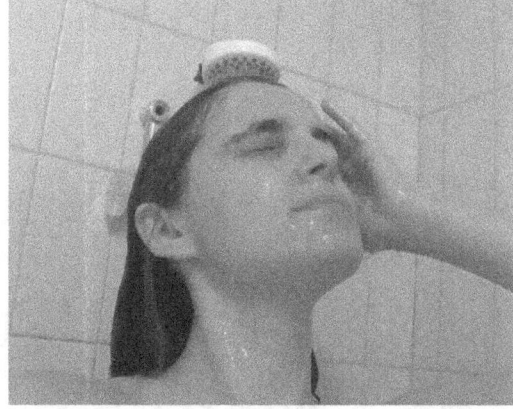

I find out they have showers and try to warm myself in hot water. The water isn't warm at all, at least not to me. I get no relief. My next attempt to get warm is to do exercises in the room. No amount of hot noodles or tea will warm me up.

Only time helps it along, which in practical terms means that I have cleared the engorgement and am getting better.

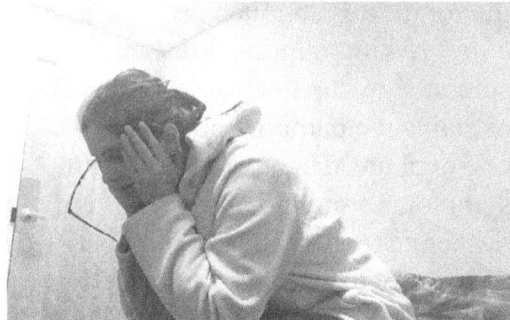

The feeding rotation is very lonely. I have not seen family at this time, and I am at almost no sleep. There is no internet access in the hospital. There is no need for anything. I'm busy.

Only now that I am writing this book I realize that this was engorgement and not a sickness. I misunderstood my symptoms.

Meanwhile, all other daily parenting activities continue: daily vitals checks, diapers, changing of clothing and baths. I start to put him on his tummy to work on muscles. Even though he is the age of a newborn, his muscles have been around four months now. I continue to read and sing to him. Basically, anything I would do at home I try to do here.

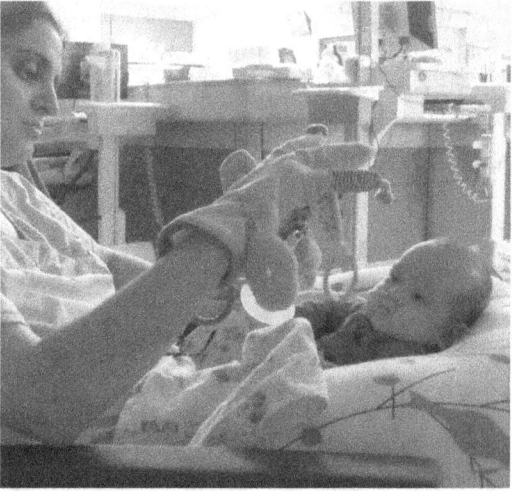

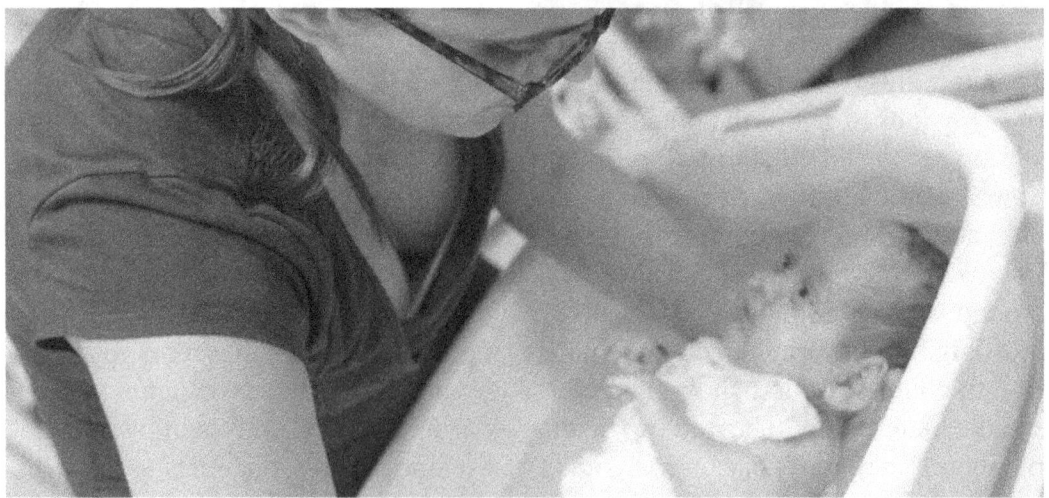

Engorgement is when you do not empty out your milk and it becomes rock like or swollen. It can lead to infections. It is painful and on my body presents flu like symptoms and even faint. Maybe faint is from stress. I have no idea.

A few days into the bunk train, they tell me to move out. They say there is no space. They talk as if they are choosing six mothers and I am not among them even though I am already IN A ROOM. They talk as if I do not exist. I am stunned. They want to give the room to other new mothers who will be gone after a couple of days. My months of work mean nothing because the quicker patients are more important to get them out of this ward and preserve the illusion that this hospital advocates breastfeeding. I pack up and vacate the room.

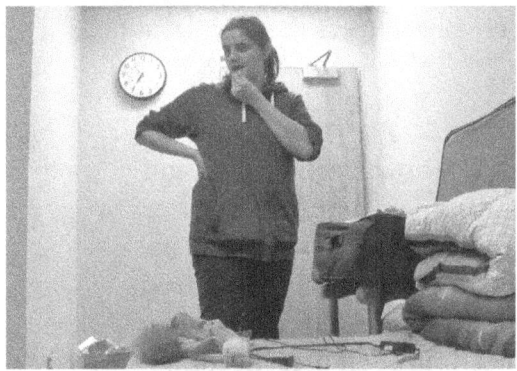

After more crying and begging, they compromise by telling me that if by chance any bunk shall open up, I can have it for that night. Meanwhile, I take my suitcase with me to Level 2 as I wait on this daily lottery for the bunk room. The plan is to sleep on the couch next to his crib if there is no bunk. My breastfeeding numbers in the first few days have been amazing. I have no reason to quit.

I bring my suitcase into the NICU with me with the hope to use what I have in there for future nights. Unaware of why I get so cold, I think that it is the unheated rooms. I keep extra blankets, a small heater and things to make food. Self-made tea to saves me money. However a nurse comes up to me and tells me that I am not allowed to keep my suitcase there. I try to explain that it is for my bunk room. It does not matter, NICUs don't allow things apart from my hand bag. It makes sense. I look around in the hospital where I can hide it but there is no place. Honestly if I just understood that the engorgement caused me to need these things I would pack less. Gosh I wish we were told about these things. I know nothing about pumping at this point. Looking at the photo below, I did bring in a lot, didn't I? I thought I was in it for the long-term... or at least two weeks.

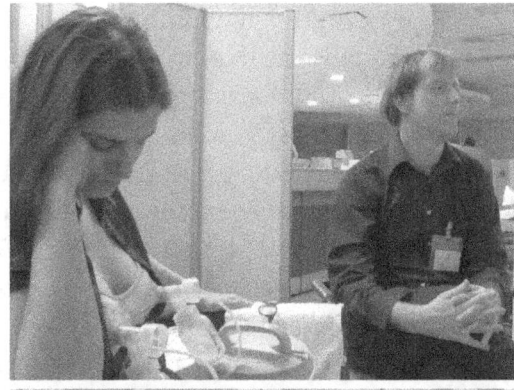

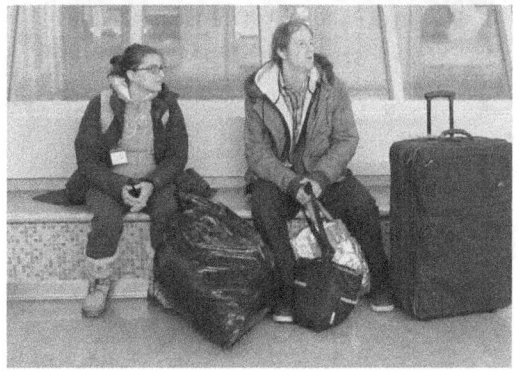

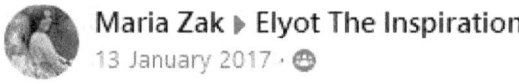

Maria Zak ▶ Elyot The Inspiration
13 January 2017

Just bumped into social worker. Here's the conversation:
SW - you have to work with us on this.
(notice how she says 'us')
Me- I am, of course I am!
Sw rolls eyes.
SW- no blankets are allowed in the NICU
Me- ok, I'll not use a blanket.

I told her I understand the bunk room needs to be shared but she refuses for me to find other ways to stay. Elyot is surprising everyone with his feeds. It's thanks to him mommy coming every 3 hours to work on it! We have momentum and just because 'it is the way it is ', I'm not accepting the present situation in it's flawed way! I am not accepting an unsupportive status quo. Of course I'll share the room to give other moms a chance. But if you have no alternatives for us then I'm creating some.

During the day, I continue to update my breastfeeding logs and see progress happening. Every now and then, a nurse sees us cry and tells me to stop and move on. Another nurse will praise me for trying. I see the posters on the walls encouraging breastfeeding – unless you have a micro-preemie – I think to myself. We are already feeding him half of his full feed through breastfeeding, and it is not even a week into the process. He eats 60ml through the tube and already managing 30ml orally. All he needs now is time to develop his stamina since he falls asleep during his feeds. He just needs time. For a couple of nights, I do get empty rooms, which means that I can fight another night. Each day I look around with the hope to find someone in charge and ask them if any rooms are open. So far I am lucky and for the next few nights I get the rooms. I find out at nine that night if it is free, sometimes later if I cannot find anyone in charge in time.

I only have my sister to rely on lifts and she is pregnant now and wakes up early for work. I try to know about the rooms as early as possible so that I do not trouble her with a late lift. If I know early enough she can bring me some stuff for the night and extra clothes to stay warm. It is a minimal bag now because in the morning I pack it all up as I say good bye to the wonderful room, and carry the bag with me for the rest of the day.

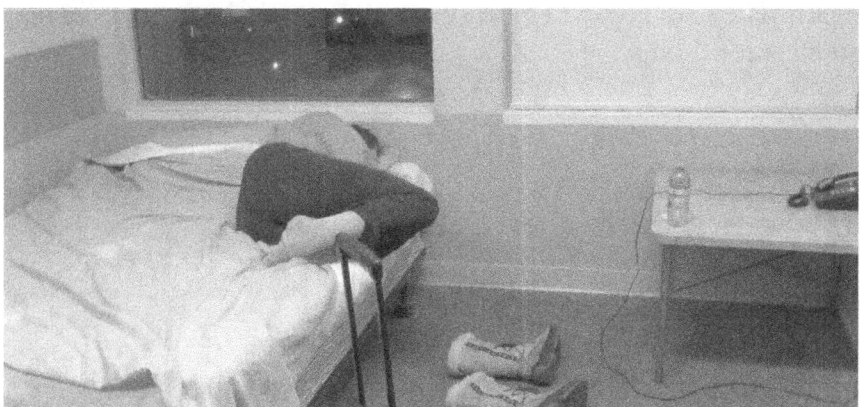

During those twelve am and three am sessions, I am the only one there breastfeeding, so I wonder who has those rooms occupied. I spend my nights crying instead of sleeping and days buying the cheapest muffins from the cafeteria to save money.

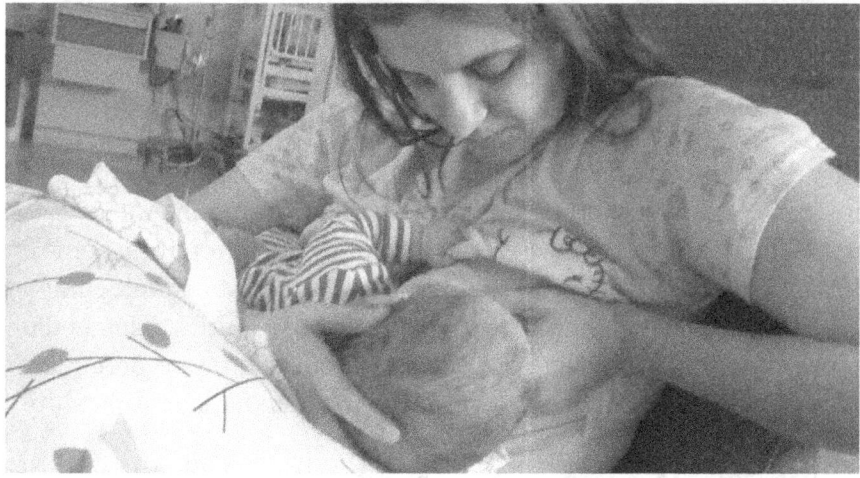

Crying Over Spilled Milk

The stress starts to do more damage. I begin to lose my milk. It is not gradual but very instant. From filling up the bottles they shrink to a third. Not only will I not be allowed to try to breast-feed, but now I might not have any milk to last till he goes since I recently donated it all and was working to rebuild my stash again. They are going to take away all his milk, but I guess bunk rooms are a luxury.

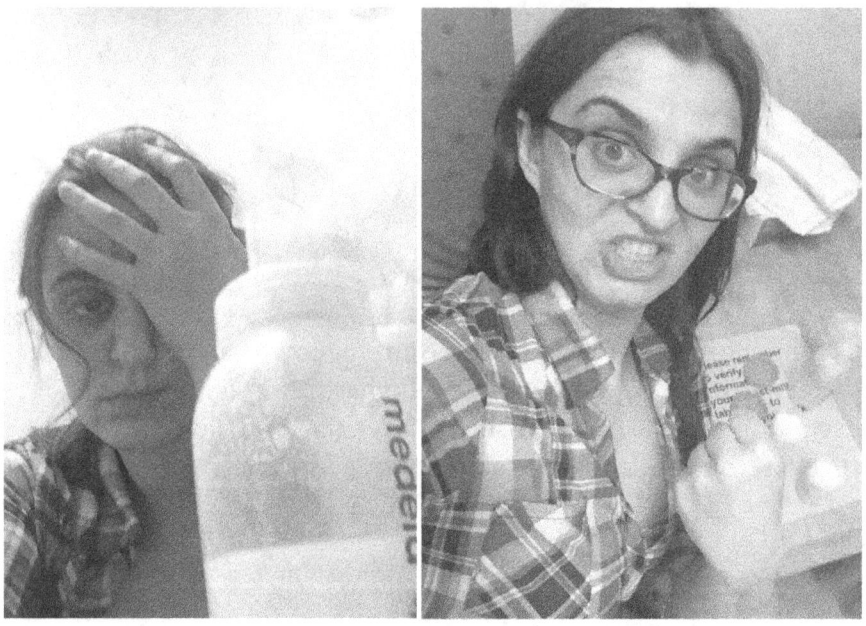

I try everything. It takes a lot of physical and emotional labour to get these bottles full again. Water ends up being the most powerful ally. Once I discover it I drink to the point of discomfort. I have never cried over milk before. It is not just a feeding resource; it is Elyot's immune system in these bottles. This is the most cruel thing that can happen to a parent of a micro preemie or sick child. It is the most cruel thing that can happen to healthy baby's as well.

  I keep this hidden from Geoff and mama because they would not be able to handle it. And thankfully each time I lose it, I always manage to bring it back.

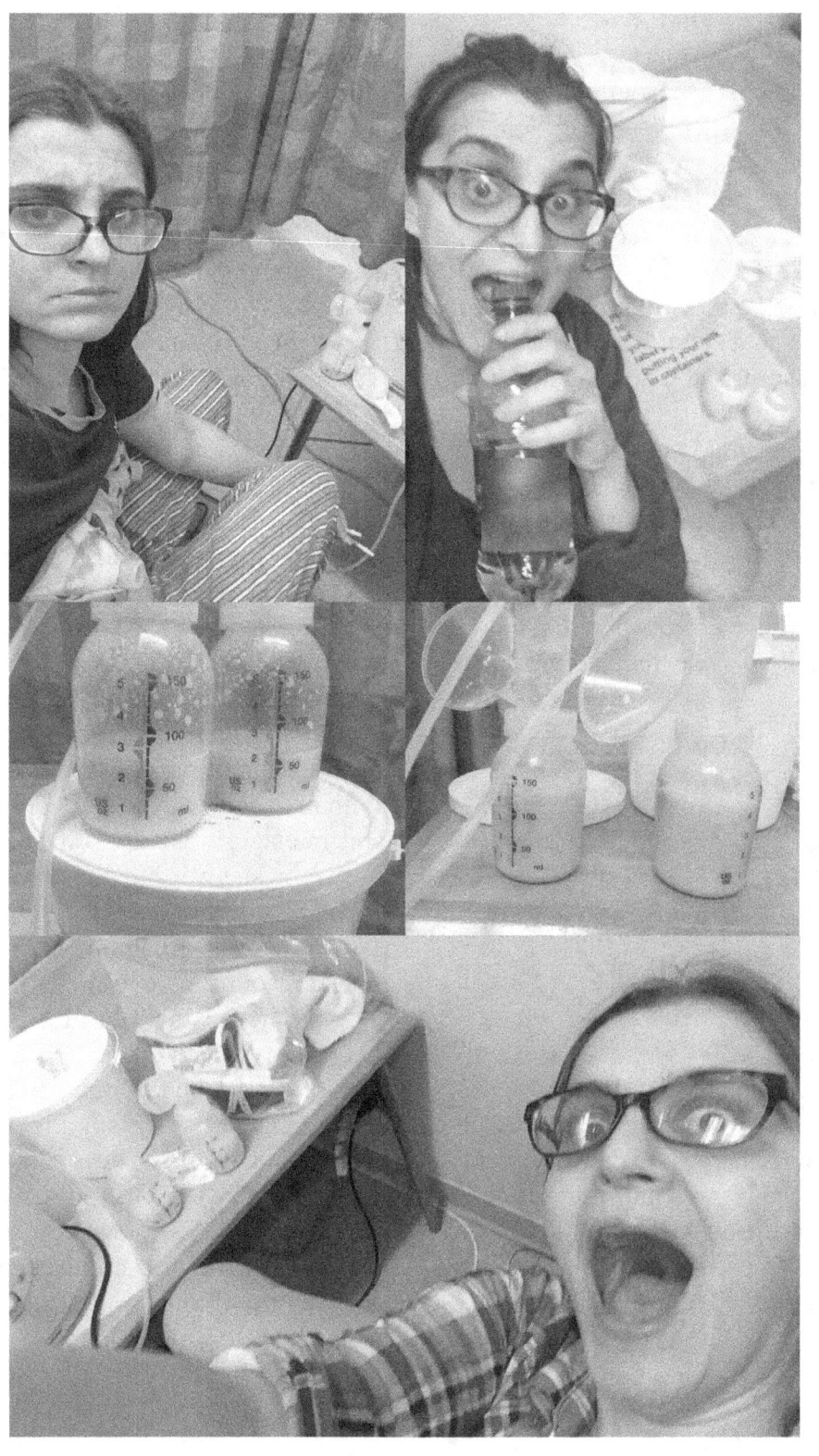

They Win

Then it happens. They tell me to try a bottle. Try it while you breastfeed; that way, he can learn to do both. Try at least one bottle a day. The bottle is already there, and everything is set up as I enter the ward. The nurse is waiting. Initially, they told me to avoid the bottle as he develops breastfeeding, so I am surprised that we can work on both. If this will speed my time out of here, then sure, I shall try. Today Elyot is going over 30ml. Tomorrow will probably be 40 ml based on where my logs are going. But I appreciate them helping me with both feeding styles so that I have a backup with the bottle eventually if breastfeeding reaches a wall.

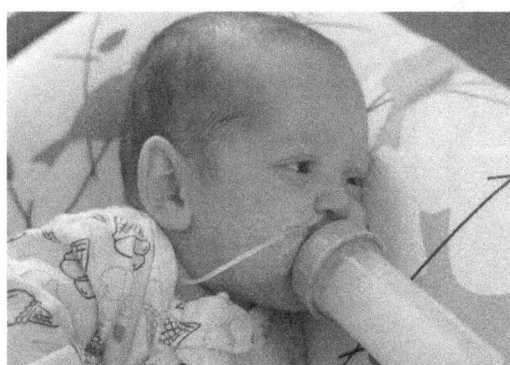

He is so cute. I enjoy the experience. I am excited to work on the bottle. Elyot chokes. He barely gets anything in. Breastfeeding was more successful. This bottle flow is too fast and stressful for him, so we feed him with his tube the rest of it. I miss a breastfeeding session.

It is a trick. We fall for it. This is our death sentence of the bunk room. The following day they tell me that we will no longer be offered me rooms. I am not exclusively breastfeeding anymore; the rooms are only for people exclusively breastfeeding. I tell them that I changed my mind, let us stop the bottle, but it is too late. Even if I never give him a bottle every again I am still considered not 'exclusively breastfeeding'. One bottle was all they needed. And yes I did it. I did it. I sat myself on my knees begging for mercy. I said the word mercy. I went full Shakespeare. When she saw me do this she abruptly turned away. Yesterday she acted like she was working with me, now she doesn't want to see my anymore. she is annoyed at me. I realize later that they probably had meetings about me and were excited to finally find a way to get rid of me. This manager was never on my side. Or maybe she was but someone higher up did this. I have no idea. To this day I am not angry at them, it is not their fault if resources are low. But I am angry at the abstract beast that Level 2 is. I have not healed from this part of the story as I type this out. My heart is racing at angry patterns. I do not want to shame the staff because I do not know their story. To the nurses who shamed me, maybe they knew more then me. Maybe they have seen my story a million times and were trying to save me from wasting time.

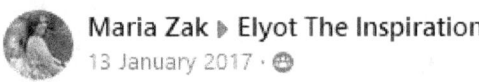

Maria Zak ▶ Elyot The Inspiration
13 January 2017

I knew this day would come but I have to have my stuff out of the bunk room. The pretend social worker was trying to convince me that it's fine skip 5 feeds or that my extended family should give me rides in the middle of the night. I told them how it's an oppressive system that doesn't care about low income women with no car. It's ok my solution is too sleep on the chair by his bedside. I told them the feeds have been improving and it's breastfeed suicide to stop the momentum. I told them how my mother advocated for me my whole life and now it's my turn to do that for Elyot. Through 4 immigrations my mother sacrificed and persevered and made it wonderful and I can do the same for Ely. We'll see what happens. They only have 6 rooms for 61 babies. I knew this would happen eventually.

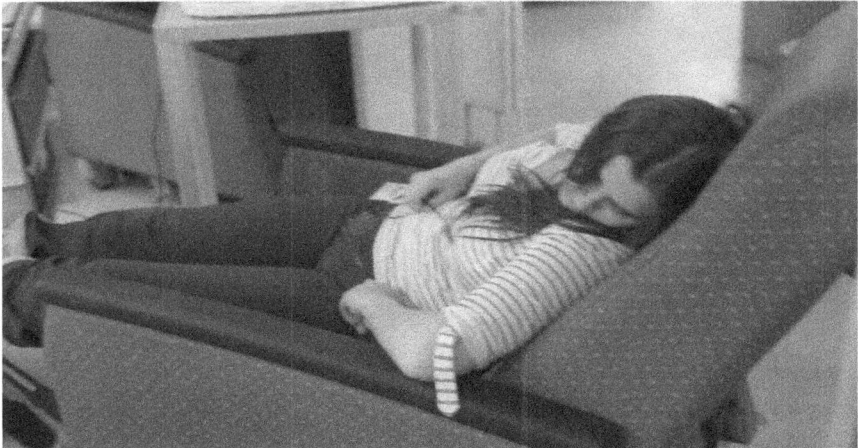

Now for Plan B. I beg them to find me a bed anywhere in the hospital, a couch. They say no. That night at nine is also his best feed yet. We are improving. I am the only one feeding at night, but it does not matter. I try to attempt to spend the night sleeping on the chair next to him. I can't fall asleep. I leave the NICU and try to lie down on benches in the common area. It is too loud. I'm suffering.

Sasha's perspective

> She just needed one more feed to motivate her. One more feed and maybe she could have lasted the first night. Instead I got woken up by a call at 1 am at night. She was sobbing. Said that Elyot slept through the feed and she had no more left to try for 3 am. No sleep had taken a toll. In her voice I heard a person giving up. I have not known her to give up anything. She knew it too, but could not fight any longer. I felt helpless.

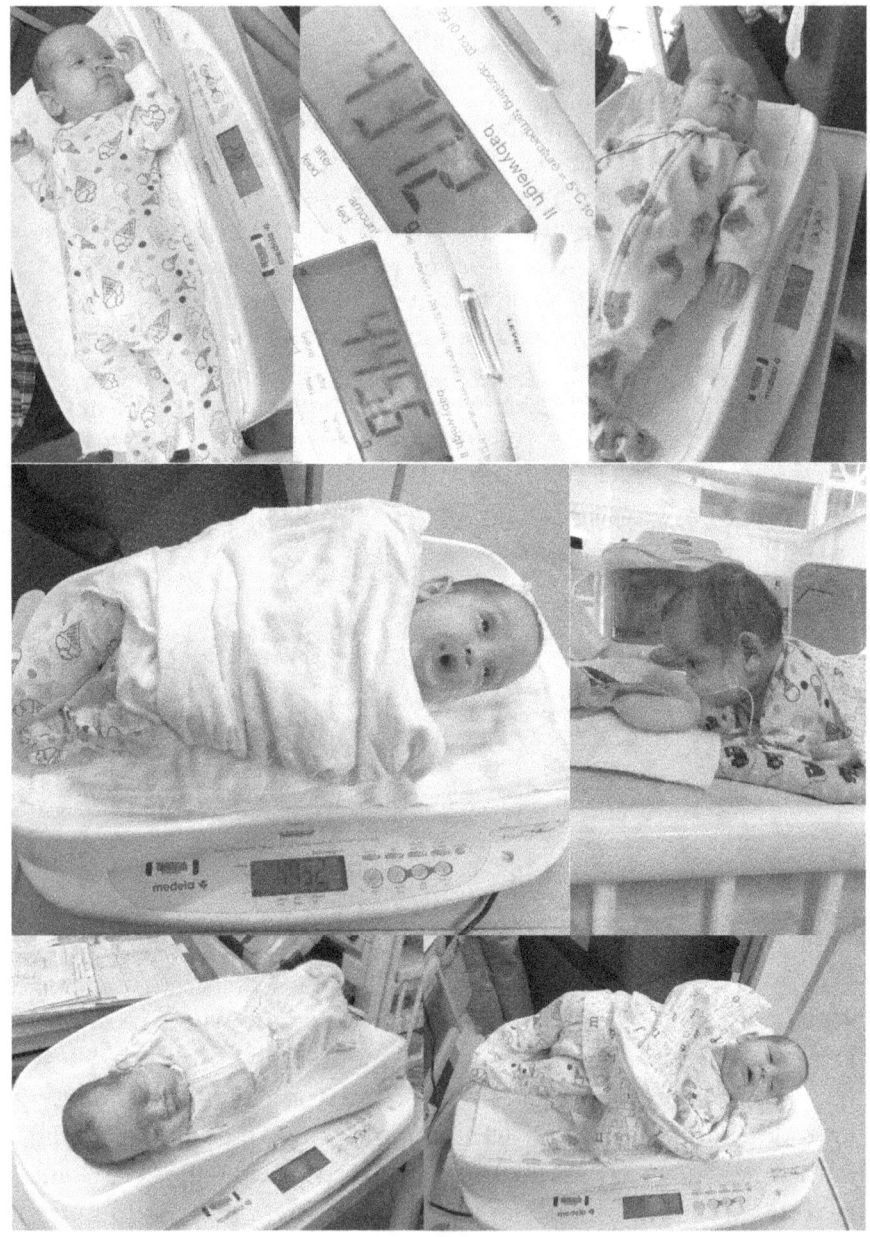

With time Elyot develops a severe colic reaction to the bottle and also a feeding trauma. We shall spend years doing feeding therapy. The bottle will damage him.

Nothing is promised at the NICU, not even a month of breastfeeding. We leave the bunk and very soon are transferred to another hospital that has no beds on offer. We leave behind our dream of breastfeeding, utterly betrayed by the same hospital with posters encouraging breastfeeding on every wall. I shall not dwell on our last days here; I just do not care anymore. Level 2 was supposed to be our happiest time but instead was a nightmare. They place him into a transport incubator, hand me an address, and off I go. There is no warning. I just found out about this, and it is happening a few hours later. I am embarrassed in front of the pitying of other parents looking at me and pretend to be excited to move finally. I am not. I feel cheated. The only positive is to leave these people who have been after me for days. I am exhausted. My fight did get me something; I am going to a less intensive Level 2 in another Hamtown hospital. Malerie did not get her to win in this one.

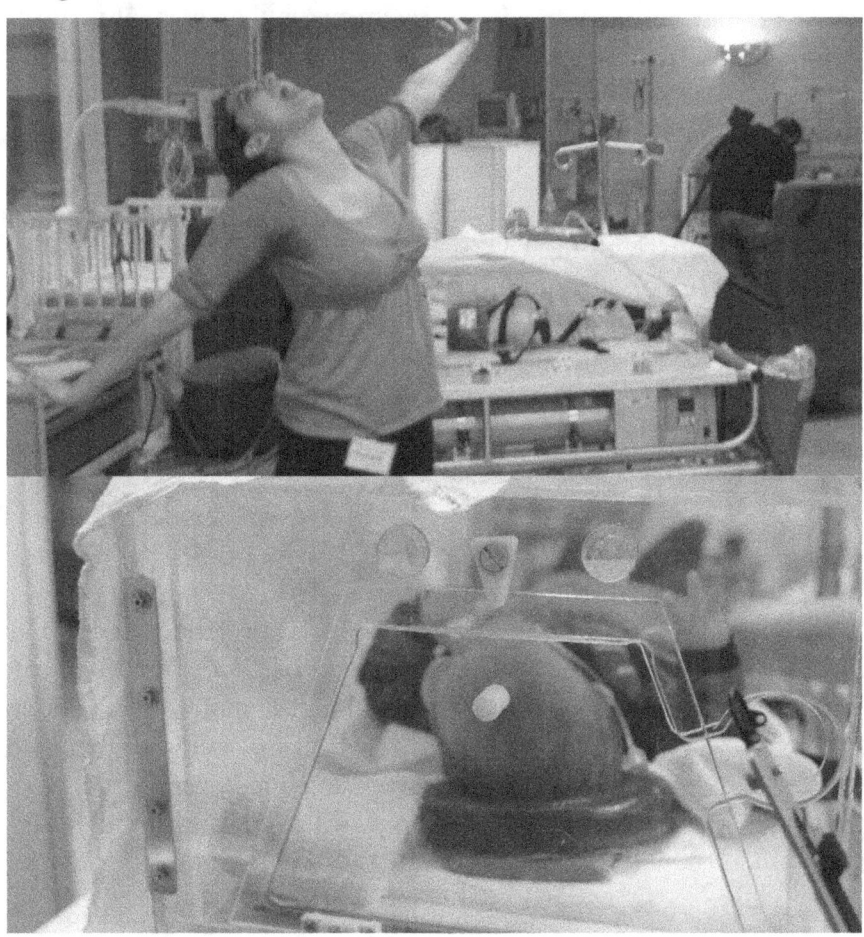

The Last Place

The minute I enter the next place, I forget my sorrows. The nurses are kind. They are cheerful, and they love Elyot. A less intense ward, they have this privilege. I am at home. This Level 2 is small. A mere whisper can travel across the room. The nurses talk among themselves and make jokes. They are less stressed here. All the babies are healthier looking. Some issues they might have are addiction or low weight, not so much because the parent had birthing complications. None of these babies stay long, and actually, this place looks relatively empty, as if there are not enough babies to fill it. I do not feel the same factory attitude here that anyone wants you out. They do a few tests to make sure Elyot is not contagious with anything, so we go through isolation again. Nothing can hurt me now. After Level 2 from the previous hospital, this place is a piece of heaven. A few days in, they offer us a private little room they created. They know how long I have been in hospital with Elyot and want to make my last stretch cozy and comfortable.

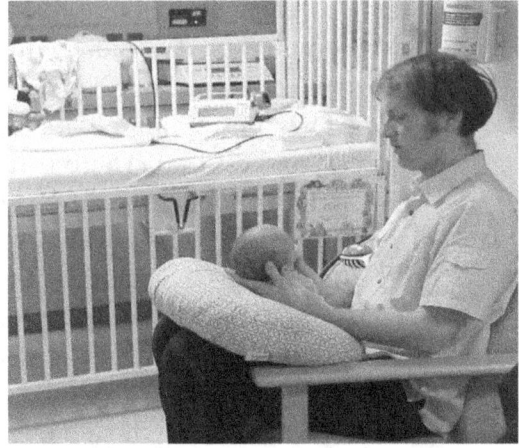

My tiny new apartment is not created by curtains but rather with walls. In here I play music, I sing, and I dance.

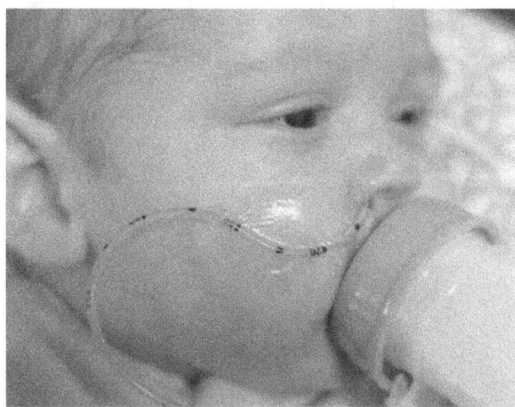

Here Elyot is not in danger and is like those other babies I envied so much; he is here to learn to feed. We do not worry about infection, heart rate or breathing. His monitor is off, and apart from his lone feeding tube, he has no wires attached to him. It is a good way to practice not to depend on knowing all of Elyot's vital scores. It prepares me for home.

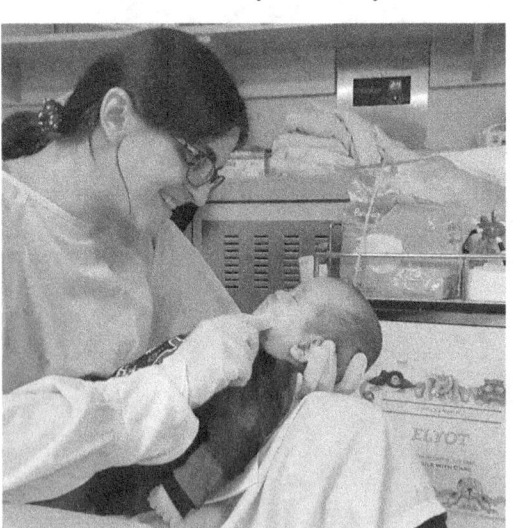

5 Months

Meanwhile, Geoff's extended family comes to visit. Elyot's cousin Ellie is not allowed in because toddlers and school children are deemed too risky with childhood diseases, including the deadly RSV. For her young years, Ellie has been keeping updates on Elyot and is utterly heartbroken when she is not allowed to see him. She falls to the floor, crying harder than I have ever seen her cry. They interact through the glass. But such is the reality of NICUs. Such shall be the reality for many places when Covid 19 happens years later. This is why we premature baby parents say that we had lived Covid 19 style lifestyle before the world got to experience it.

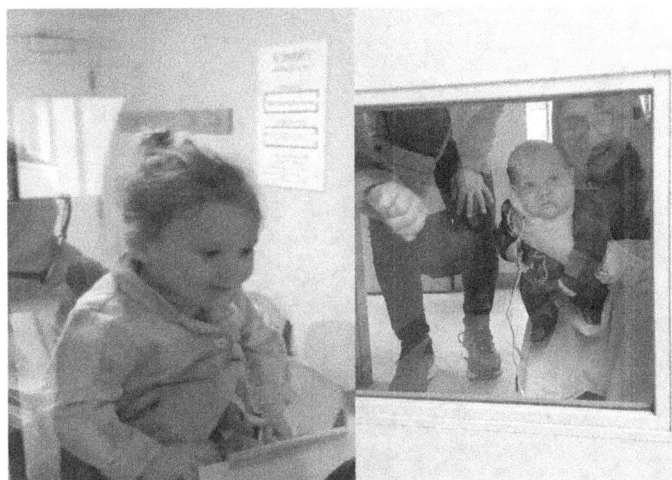
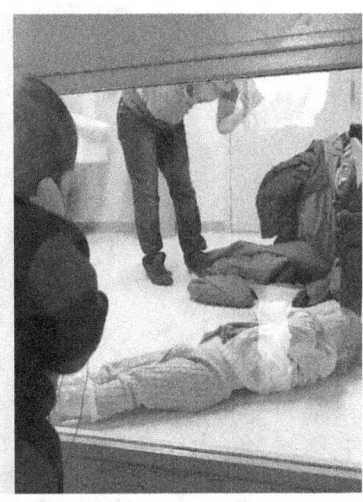

This last stretch might be the hardest part of the NICU. It does not have the intensity of Level 3 NICU to distract you; it does not have the fighting spirit of Level 2 breastfeeding. All we have left now is pure waiting for Elyot to learn to feed without a tube. We are counting the millilitres of each bottle. His lungs are weak, and he has no stamina for drinking. The goal is to spend several days entirely off the feeding tube.

One of the nurses looks at him and says, "I better not see you here by Valentine's Day." She looks at me and makes me a promise that I shall be home for Valentine's. Here they make promises!

They make promises! They are not afraid. We are no longer in the intensive world of sick babies; here, all babies go home. None of this nothing is promised philosophy.

Newborn Photography

Days are long. Apart from daily chores, I have nothing to do. The truth is that time has never been slower. As mentioned earlier, the faster time passes within these pages, the slower it is in real life because of how identical each day is. I discover that the crib has a great spotlight over it that is probably for medical procedures. My time to do newborn photography has arrived. I set up a whole studio. Elyot has been around for over five months now but is still a newborn, a chubby newborn with full head support and strength of older babies. But a newborn still.

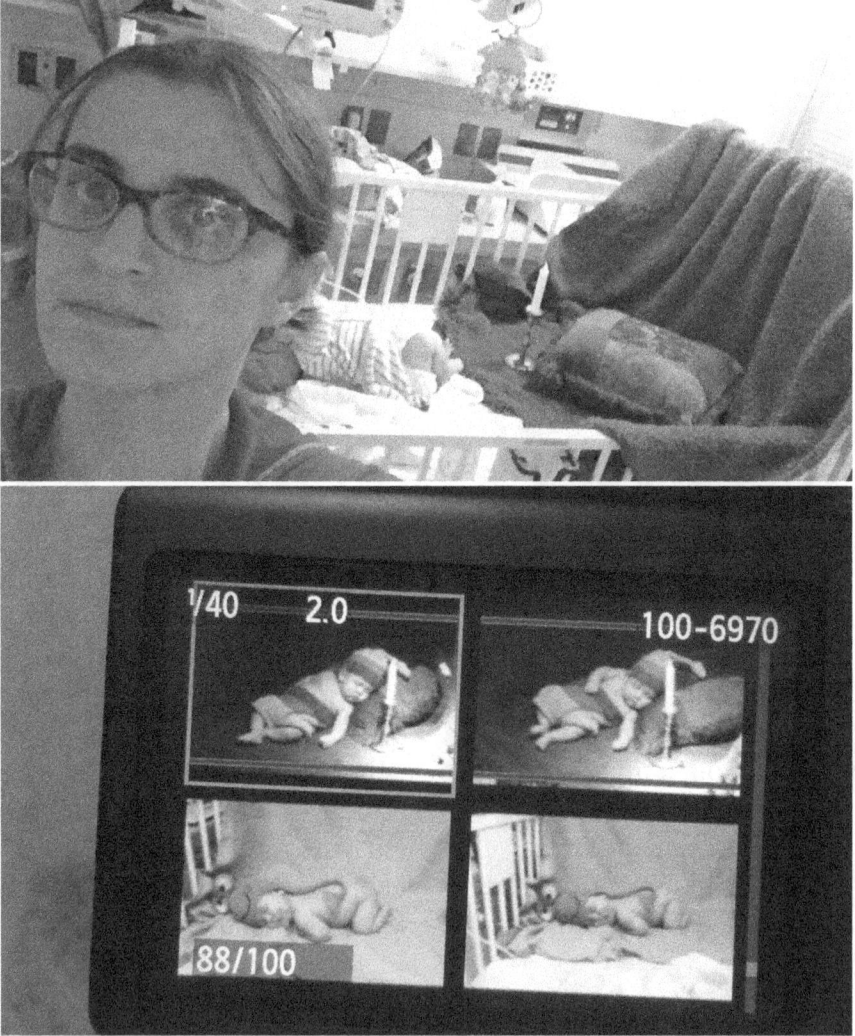

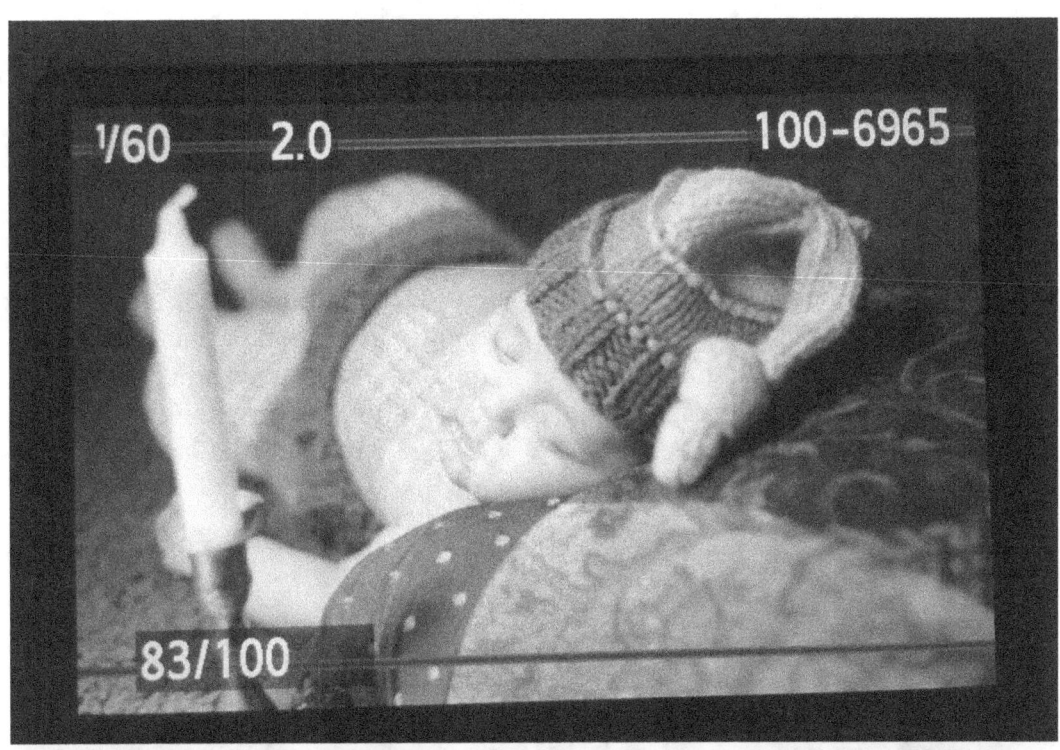
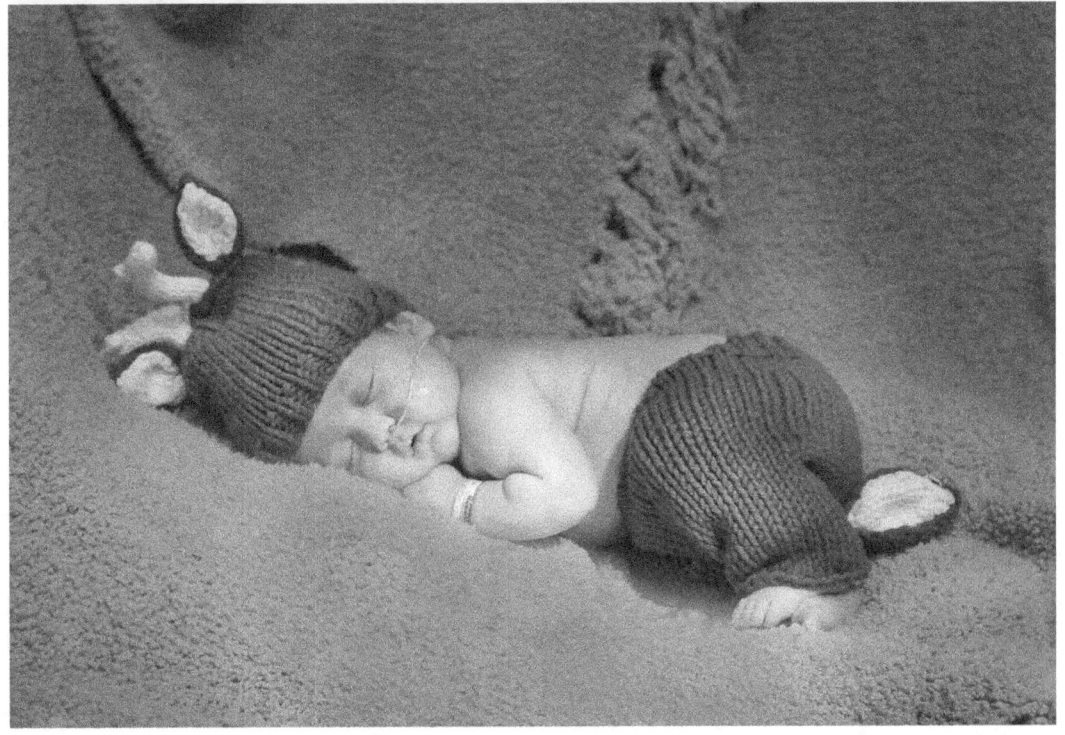

Like Home

I feel free here. I have new portable pumps and just walk around this relaxed ward. Besides helping with feeds, no one checks up on me. For the first time, Elyot gets to see outside the window. We talk about the world and our plans for the future.

Elyot is struggling with the bottle. He did much better with breastfeeding; the flow was slower and gentler on him for the pace that he needed. The bottle is more aggressive, so he is out of breath and exhausts in most feeds. He is scared of the faster flow of the nipple on the bottle and takes time to adjust to it. It is because he is not a regular newborn but a micro-preemie with a lung history. Another problem is gas. He won't burp. He suffers from the bottle. It is another micro-preemie symptom you discover to be unable to burp it out. We are living this now. There are days when he has no feeds at all.

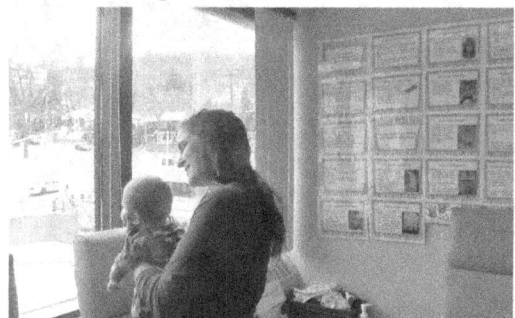
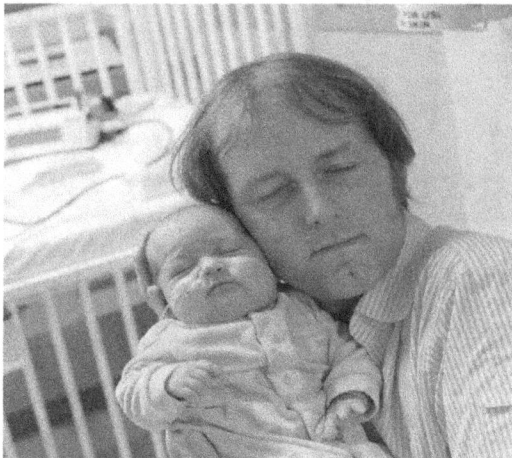
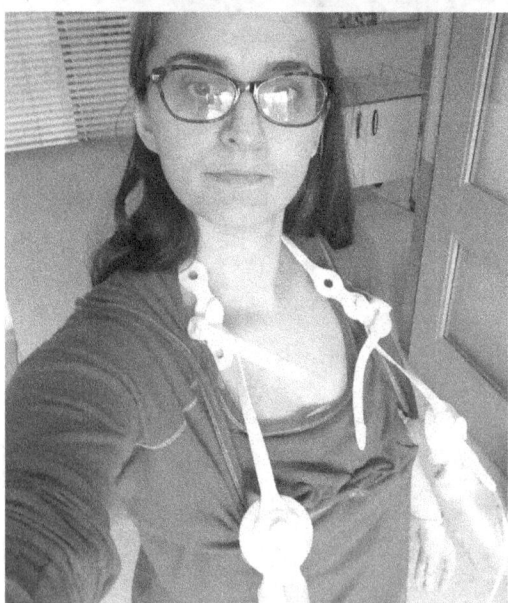
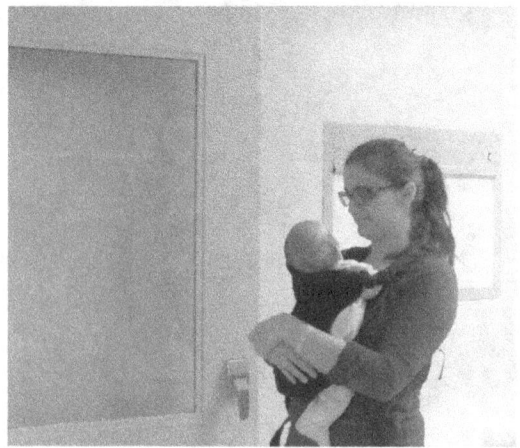

Otherwise, it is almost a copy of a home as we fold his clothes for the day, do baby wearing in the corridors and his tummy time exercises. This is why it is so important to be at the right hospital. Had I been in Yorkton, I would have seen Geoff more often but would have had no other family help me. Here in Hamtown, I have both him though he travels far to see us, but I have daily family members help me. My in-laws and my sister's in-laws and friends. Overall Hamtown is the place to be. Had the social worker had her way, I would be in a faraway city with no one. I would arrive late and go home early. Here I get lifts so I can be here with him all day long.

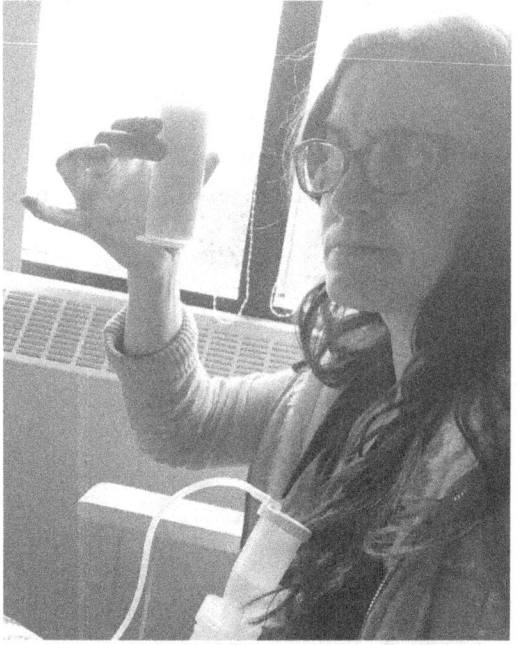

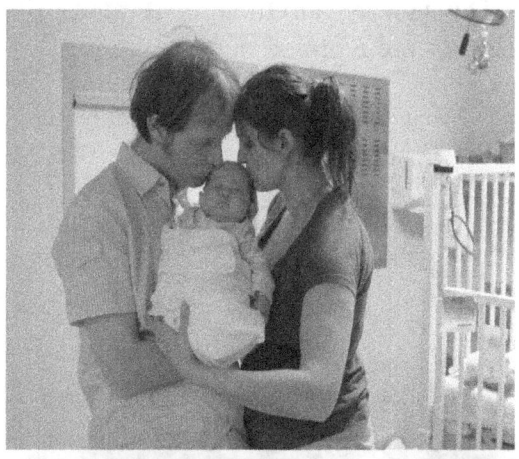

Also, all my milk is back. Being back to a proper routine and less stress because no one is threatening us anymore, I have returned it all to its former glory and start to save my stash again.

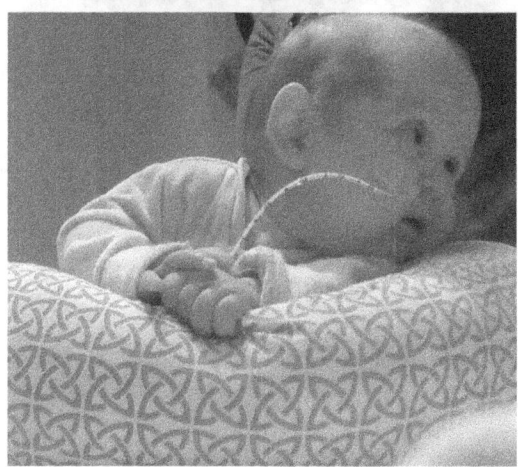

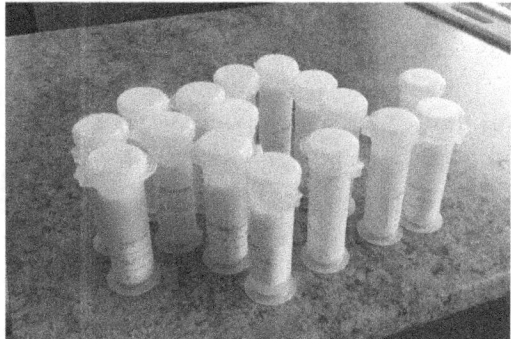

6 Months

The Face with No Tubes

What is a mere next page here is a month worth of work in reality. Today he pulled his tube off, and the nurses do not rush to replace it. His skin has been torn on both cheeks where it was taped because of the times he pulls it. Keeping it off will give him some time to heal.

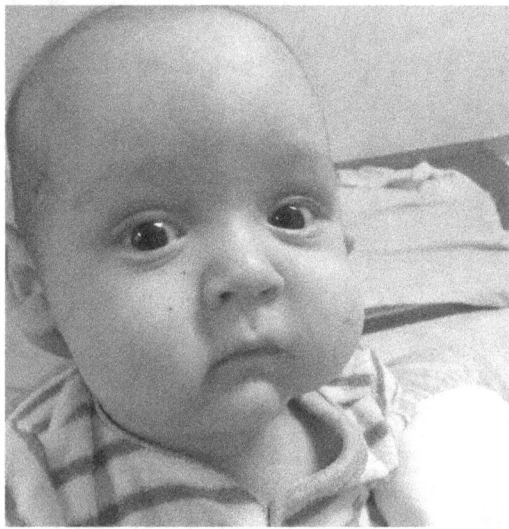

The idea these days is to keep the tube off until it is needed. He is slowly getting stronger to stay awake during his feeds, and lately, he has a few full bottles in a row. At night the nurses do the feeds. They also work to train him to be a night sleeper for me when I take him home.

So many subtle gestures of love come from these nurses. He is a toy here, when I walk into the ward, there is always someone playing with him. Looking around in a nurse's arms. Promising. I can dwell on all his cute parts now. The nurses remind me from where I came. Not in that he is a micro-preemie, so 'life is hard' way, but in that – I am a hero who worked for six months to save my boy way.

Days go by, and the tube remains off. Bottles are emptied one by one.

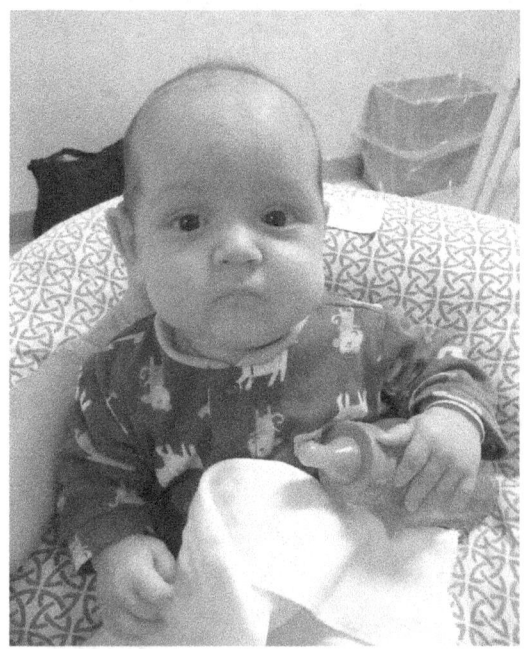

 31 January 2017

Noooooooooooo! He was 1 or two feeds away from 48 hours. But couldn't waking up for this forced on feed. He has to last 48 hours off the tube to be put onto on demand feeding. Laughing in his sleep too!

Care By Parent Room

It is not the same as the previous bunk room. It is just a random empty bed within the Maternity Ward, something the last hospital said they do not have. It is only for final days to prove that parents can do this independently, not learn to breastfeed or any other skills. I have less bitterness about not breastfeeding because I just want to go home, and tonight I have to prove to them I can feed him for a 24-hour cycle with a bottle. Or more so, Elyot has to prove that he can do it. We are both on display tonight. The nurses are so encouraging that I do not know if I shall do the work for myself or just to make them happy.

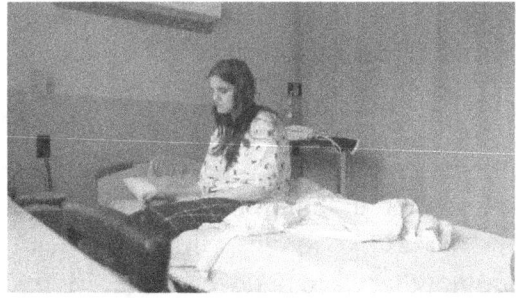

finish most of his bottles. He is sleepier than any other time recently that I have seen him.

Wake up, Elyot! Please wake up. It is such a desperate plea. I have unwashed pumps back in the room and premixed tiny bits of formula to fortify the milk. They want him to gain more calories, so I add formula to the milk. I just do not understand this fortifying stuff. Elyot is already so chubby.

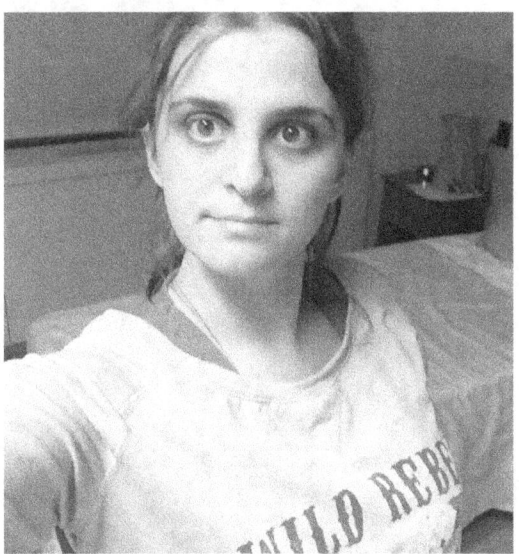

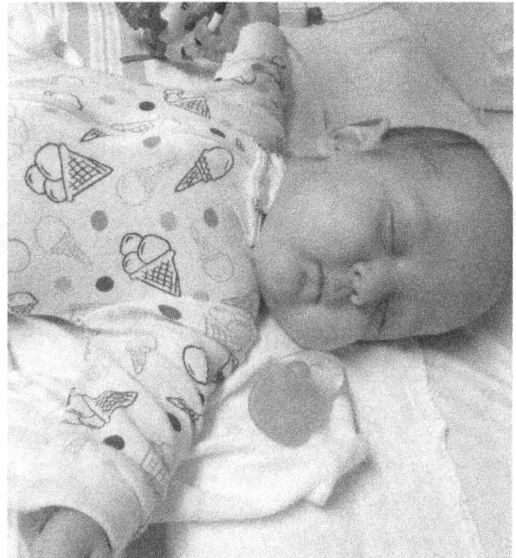

We start the process apart where I go in to feed him every three hours on the first night. I have no memory of that first night. The only evidence I have are photos taken at that time. He does not

However, in the morning, the nurses are actually happy with the result. Unexpectedly they consider it a success, and we organize another night of this schedule. I do this for two nights.

The cafeteria downstairs is expensive big meals only, so I avoid it. There is a coffee shop, but by now, I am so sick of everything there. This hospital is further away, so I have fewer people able to visit me and help me with Elyot. Sasha is at work. I am entirely alone here. However, if I do get some extra sleep in the morning, I know that the nurses like to play with him when I am not there. He is never alone. Elyot might not go home this week, but it is getting close. I just know it.

Geoff joins me at night from Yorkton and returns to work in the mornings. He takes with him his sleeping bag and blow up mattress back to work on the train. On the first night, Elyot pretty much sleeps through the whole night. Only I am up pumping, I realize looking back that the nurses sleep trained him, that us why he sleeps and does not eat at night.

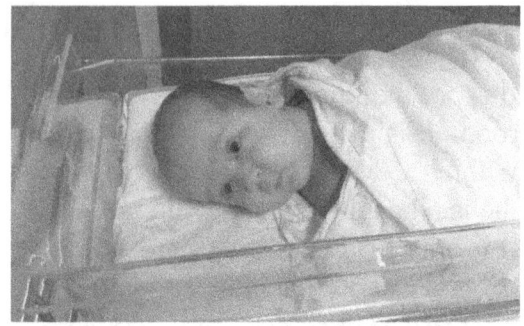

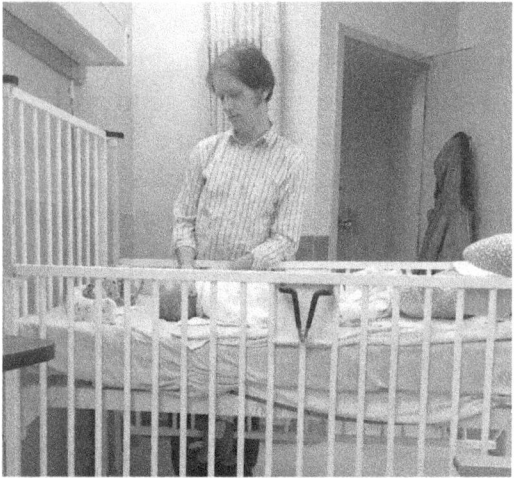

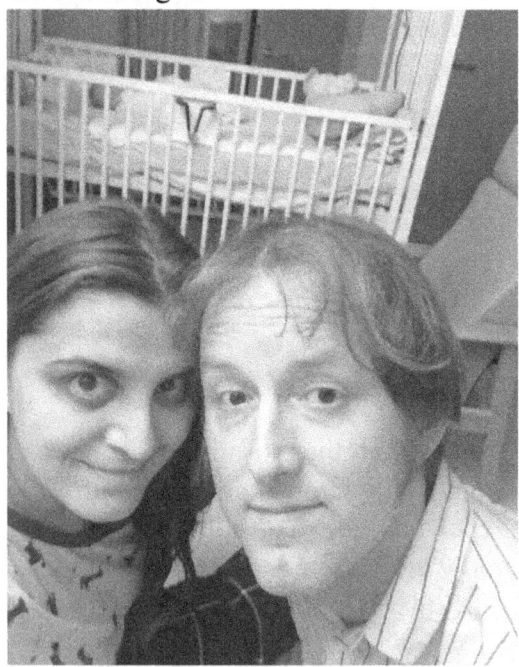

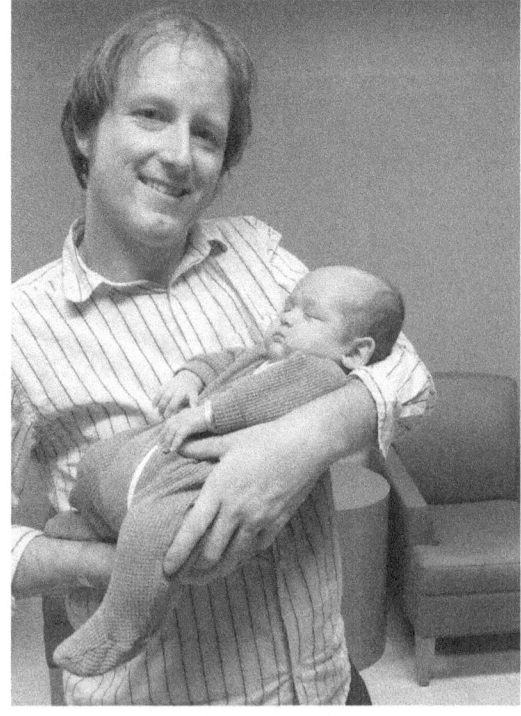

We cart him around in this glass container. It feels wonderful to be mobile together. Notice he still has a bit of an egg shape head from the C PAP mask. It is going away but is still there today. We are now those families whom I envied in the previous Level 2. They were among the most stressed-out parents I have seen. They live off a different schedule than the long-term families. Their pace is faster; their voices are louder. They just want to rush home. I understand them now because babies do not always cooperate,. However, within a few days or a week, they all go home excited and ready for their new lives. I know that our time might be adjusted by a few days, but it shall happen very soon.

And meanwhile as we have breakfast together Geoff brought me some fruit fusion tea like the old times. A romantic and symbolic gesture that we are going to get our 'normal' back.

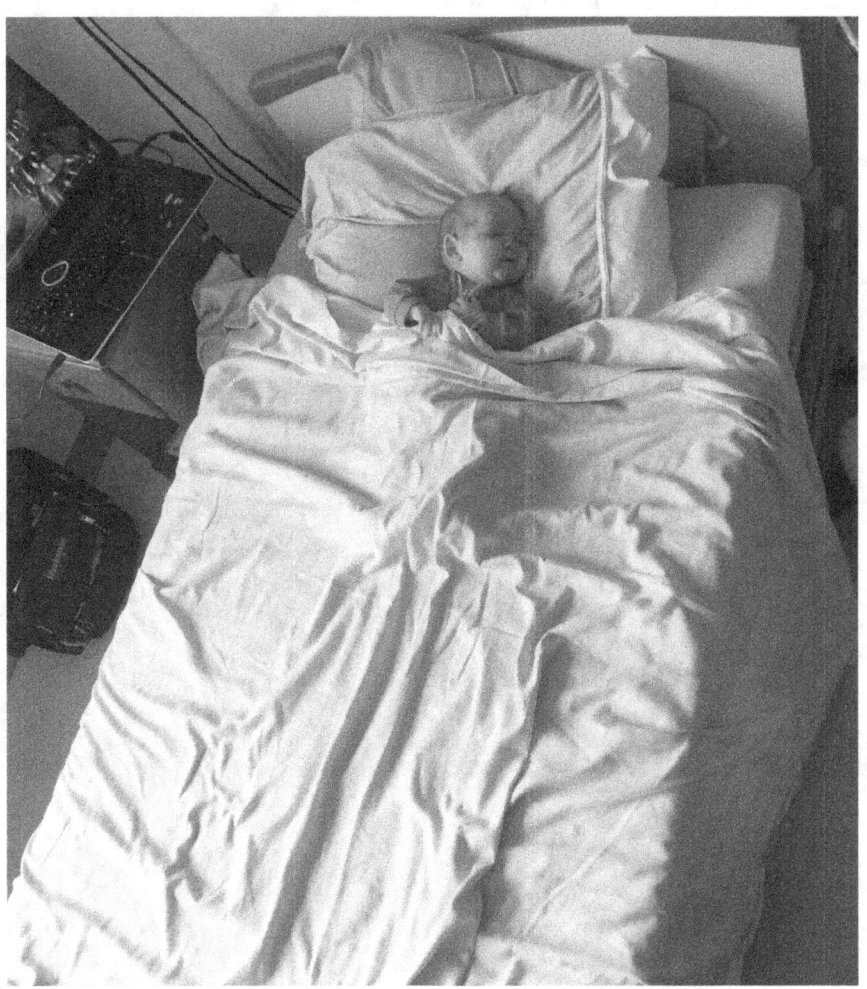

That fourth morning after our anxious roaming around the hospital, Geoff is now gone to work, and I do the slow walk to the NICU. The nurse greets me with high energy and tells me that Elyot is doing very well, to call family to be ready to pick us up because after the paperwork is done, we can go home. It feels so surreal, like they are going to change their minds.
The NICU is empty; no other babies, no nurses are in the room at the time. Just Elyot and myself with all the equipment as we say goodbye to this unexpectedly warm place. It is a great way to end a seven-month journey from the maternity ward to here.

I take my final milestone photo of us being in jail, looking out behind bars.

We place Elyot into the car seat with no tests needed. They assume his lungs are car seat safe; Thankfully, Elyot is very strong and healthy as he leaves this place. We have a routine eye test the following day but as outpatients.

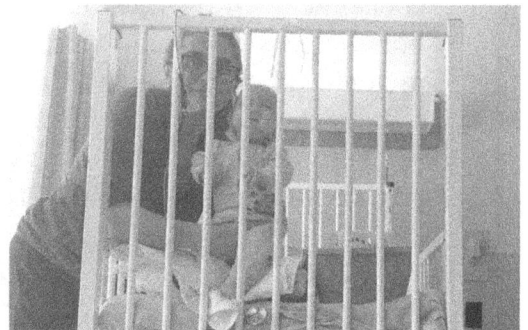

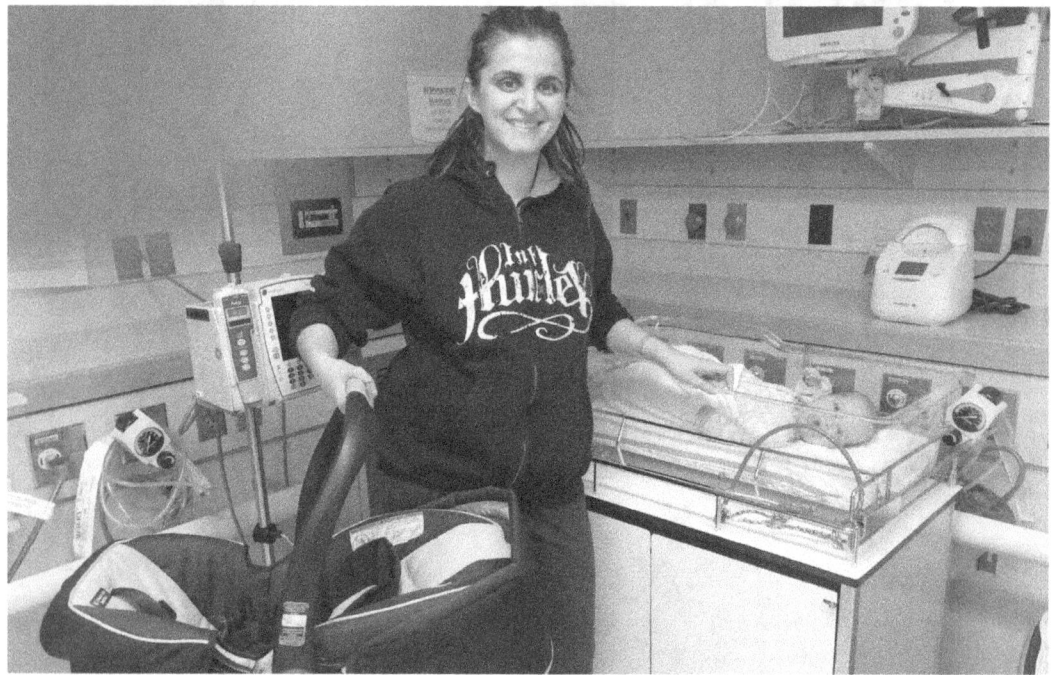

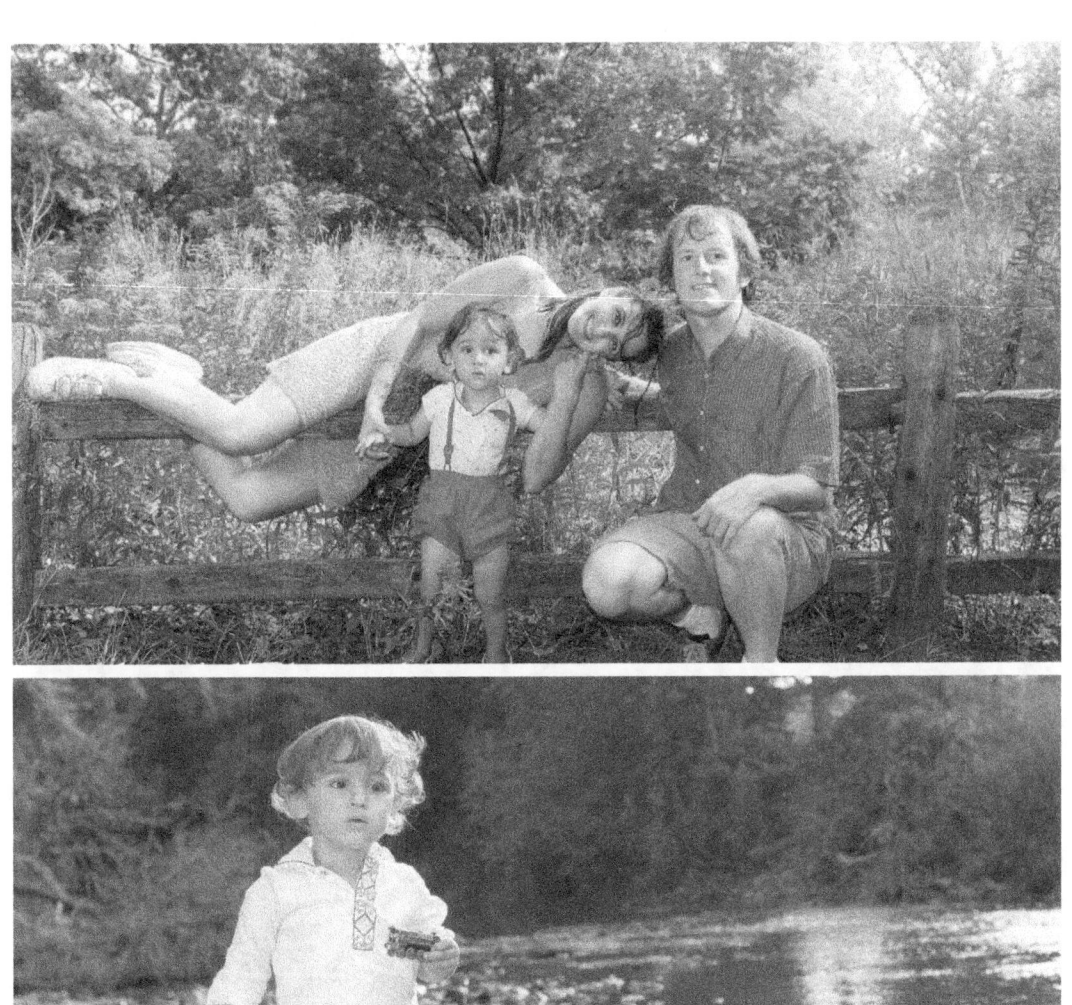

Chapter Five
Life After Hospital

"I'm too exhausted to educate, sometimes I just want to be a parent."

She texted this to me one day as she sat waiting to meet a new paediatrician.

Maternity Ward mothers and NICU parents are already part of an invisible class of people. What we had not expected was how bad it would get after the hospital. The purpose of this chapter is to have a bit of a discussion and maybe lessen the load for her to keep educating. How about I take over with this one and let Maria be 'just a parent' for once, even when she's writing a book about it. Her main intention for this book is to make sure their story is out there and becomes as common place as any other story. This includes life after the hospital.

Thanks Sasha!!!

Lets start from the beginning. Once a micro preemie always one, as they would say.

First Six Months

Elyot spent his first six months of life outside the womb fed intravenously with a tube going straight into his stomach. He was not fed on demand. He had a more scientific rigid way of eating. His feedings were on a pre-set timed schedule, with pre planned amounts. He did not have a say whether he was hungry, nor whether he has had enough. As a result he didn't learn the associations between hunger and feedings. There was no pairing with satiation and a feeding coming to an end. He has no need to develop stamina for eating. No need to be awake. He even missed out of learning how to have feeding stamina. He lost this milestone, as well as, understanding what food is. When finally he was bottle fed in Level 2 he struggled with the faster flow of the silicone nipple. They did not give them the time they needed to develop his feeding more organically.

At Home

The minute they left the hospital they had a list of appointments lined up. A routine eye test, and RSV shot and others I'm not aware of. As a micro preemie in Canada he was allowed free shots during his first RVS season for the first year of his life. Their developmental clinic was booked six months away.

When she left her home, she carried boiling water in a flask and would warm it up right there on that bus hoping not to spill it on anyone. She also would cover up his stroller in case of any germs. You're reading this book during or after Covid 19, so I can use this as a comparison. Maria's and Geoff's life in those days was very much life of Covid 19. Anything, but particularly RSV could be deadly for Elyot. They would sanitize everything, stay away from stores and remain isolated from other people in case if someone was infected. Buses were particularly stressful with people coughing.

***

At the doctor's office Maria had developmental charts to fill out. Elyot was technically much younger than the age written there. The almost four months prematurity was very confusing as to where Elyot was supposed to fit. There was no special attention paid to Elyot by anyone. He was growing well, good weight and because he had no brain bleeds at any point they didn't see the purpose to follow him extra closely. None of her doctors understood Maria's concerns whenever she asked about micro preemie issues. As long as the developmental chart showed nothing of concern no one bat an eye lash.

" I thought his micro preemie will follow him for a while? But they don't know that he is one in these appointments. Am I missing something? When did he get un-preemied?" This was the basis of many of my conversations with Maria.

***

Elyot didn't know how to burp. Micro preemies have this difficulty. He was constantly gassy and uncomfortable. Maria tried every technique to burp him but nothing was helpful. He would often cry or fuss after meals. Also Elyot would only drink milk at a specific temperature. It had to be pretty warm, much warmer than fresh milk or room temperature. It was hard to go out with him, because when he was fed he needed this warm milk to resemble the NICU's. They had to carry a bottle warmer with them everywhere they went. This meant that if he was crying and hungry on the bus and the milk cooled down a tad, there was nothing they could do until they got home.

Memory: Elyot is crying. We stop the car at a nearest plaza and Geoff runs out of the car in search of hot water. He runs into any coffee shop, a Tim Horton's, anywhere who may offer hot water to warm up the milks. Maria and I are sitting in the car anxious hoping that a kind hearted soul will say yes. It's always a gamble. Eventually he emerges with boiling water. But it takes a few minutes for his meal will be warmed up. After many repeated experiences of pleading for boiling water, Maria and Geoff catch on to needing to buy a flask. Their anxiety decreases and they gain power of heating his meals during outdoor trips. The rigid presence of his milk temperature, unfortunately, is a taught habit. It was the bi product of the hospital experience, and it was all Elyot knows and accepts. He wasn't given a chance to try hot or cold, or to not finish a feed. His habits are laid out for him, and he was a passive participant.

First Two Years

Maria was obsessed with milestones in the internet. She would look up what is expected of the next age group and practice them with Elyot before their next appointment.

"Object passed from one hand to another. He isn't doing that!"

" He isn't clapping!" "We need to stack three blocks!"

Even in the rare Developmental Clinic where Maria thought she would get advice, but he made it through without concerns. That was not an accurate picture of him because none of this came for free. Nothing was automatic. Almost every milestone he had was individually targeted by Maria and trained. The charts did not reflect the struggle or that no milestones came on their own, that she had to work hard on teaching them all.

One concern that Maria shared with them is his feeding seemed to be problematic. The Developmental Clinic said it was a pincer problem so Maria worked hard to developing his fingers. Elyot didn't have any problems with his fingers or fine motor skills.

By his first year, Elyot had not progressed from first stage baby food. It's at this point Maria realized how alone she is with having a former micro preemie. None of the doctors believed her about the feeding issues. Also, even though he just barely made it with his three words to pass his developmental assessment Maria knew that it wasn't enough. His language was stuck where it was and pretty much non-functional. His non-verbals, on the other hand were great. Maria began to invent games they could play. She put his favourite items into a box and would take them out one by one and label them. Elyot didn't have the words, but he started to understand them when she labelled them. "Car! Croc! Baba!" Elyot loved that pink croc.

"Boys are slow." "He's a micro preemie, he'll get there." "He looks great in this chart." " It's all in your head."
The worst gas-lighting came from people around her. Her friends and some extended family told her that she is torturing Elyot. Someone told her that she is killing his spirit by trying to teach him. She was bullied when she tried to give Elyot harder food. "Let him reach that stage himself!" But by the age of 24 months Elyot had never touched his face with a food item. He would chew toys but never a food item. He had never picked up any food to play with it. Not a wet food, not a dry one. He knew the difference between a real strawberry and a toy one. He rejected the real one. Wouldn't have it near him. "Let the boy have a break!" was how a lot of people responded until she stopped sharing and only showed her work to my family and me. But none of her therapies were 'work' to Elyot. They were games, toys and quality time. She was the only parent in the playground getting dirty with her baby in the sandbox. She was the only parent in mommy groups who was on the floor with Elyot showing him how cars crash while other mommies socialized with each other. It was work, but only to Maria, all Elyot experienced was a very dedicated mother.

"Babies at 12 months play with water!" She'd tell me. "Elyot doesn't see it at all." At home she would create water basins all over the house with fun things, risking spilling. The tiny apartment became a treasure trove of different toys and sensory games. Her goal was to make Elyot wake up to the world and to love it; and also to actually have the skills to enjoy it.
Very slowly Elyot started to notice them and the joy that would

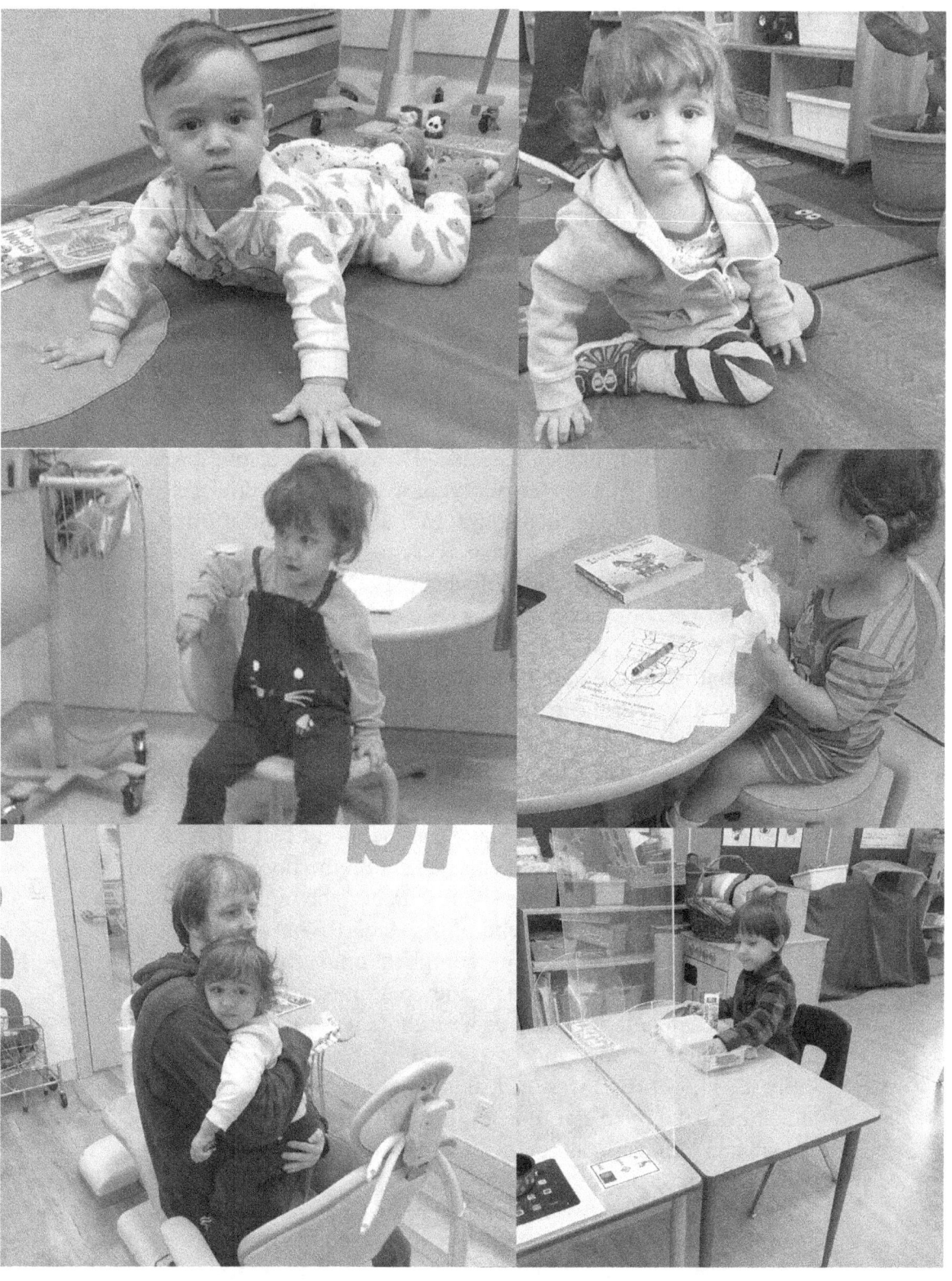

follow. Even his laughter started to change to a more belly laugh as he watched things tumble. Eventually when he saw water is when his language started to pick up. It was very much like a Hellen Keller moment. Maria turned off the tap in the bath and Elyot got upset. "Vada! Vaaaa, vaaaaaa!". Vada is water in Russian. Suddenly Elyot's cute whimper of a voice said vah! And so began their playful journey towards language. Alongside it followed other games for cognitive, social and physical.

***

Their little family has been socially and medically isolated. In the second year they had more confidence to go shopping and even had tiny coffee shop visits. But mostly stayed at home. Geoff was showing signs of real trauma. He would question anyone who got close to Elyot, even snap at friends. " Do you have a sore throat? Did you sanitize? Why is Elyot crying, what did you do?" He was pretty rude to people in those days. Maria was drawing further into isolation. I made sure to visit every weekend and help her with everything. My parents did what they could from afar. However Maria was not lonely, nor was she even depressed. She was too busy to feel any of that.

She eventually completed her Master degree. Her father in law agreed to babysit in those days. Towards the end Elyot got infected with RSV. By now Elyot was over a year and death was not so scary, rather it was a hospital stay situation. Maria completed her Master degree from within the pediatric ward. She continued all her games with Elyot and made sure he didn't feel isolated in there. She brought out a blanket, spread it on the floor and played played played with the games she researched the night before to help with speech. By the end of the week Elyot was able to return home but with one major complication. He was unable to eat anything! Nothing. The mask they put onto his face caused even more damaging trauma, as a result he was too scared to have anything touch his face.

Elyot's loss of food was critical and put him at risk for hospitalization and maybe a G tube to get nutrition in. They hired a speech and language pathologist (SLP) to return his eating and with it they added speech therapy. Maria was so happy that finally someone believed her. She started to work on both language and returning trust to eat. "Run run run jummmmp!" for words and "Bubbles pop pop!" for food. But now she had a name for it. It was a language delay and oral trauma. Now she could research games and target the skills directly.

Physical and Cognitive

Elyot was delayed with all things physical so we took him to parks to teach him to climb. We tried to make him walk up hill to work on the muscles. For cognitive Maria would give him puzzles and make funny noises when his pieces fit or didn't. Elyot loved it and laughed so hard. That was his eureka moment for cognitive. He loved it when Maria acted like a clown with him. I'm a behaviour specialist. I did more targeted play with him. I taught him to play in the playground, to notice the swings and slides. I taught him imaginative play and how to play.

Together

On the side story of all this we were successful with the Canadian immigration process and to get my parents to move here. Now they live their lives to support Elyot. It took me seven years of trying through tears. Back in Boston their delayed their retirement to get Elyot more money and end up giving all their lifesavings to get Elyot his expensive supports.

Even after Maria got her master's degree, it's fruitless. She can't use it. She stays home to teach and provide him with everything he needs. It was impossible to enrol him in daycares with his needs, particularly with his low immune system. Now in 2021 he has entered his senior kindergarten class and is caught up academically. He still struggles with speech and feeding and those will be his longest journey yet. However cognitively and physically has been fully caught up by the age of five. Now Maria can relax a bit and return her artistic hobbies that she neglected (including writing this book) and maybe one day will actually return to work, even if only part time. However long she will need to be with Elyot she will.

Feeding Issues

This issue is so big that it needs its own moment. What the doctors didn't notice is that Elyot had oral trauma from all the tubes in the NICU. Also his bottle drinking was stressful because he didn't like the fast flow even from the slowest bottle nipples.

He had severe colic and cried between all his meals. We will never know if breastfeeding would have helped him. It was his happiest time. Meanwhile Elyot missed all his baby feeding milestones and didn't learn how to use his mouth. He had weak oral motors and didn't use his tongue. Maria researched oral issues from the internet and found that the Down Syndrome and Cerebral Palsy communities had the best exercises. She ordered all the chew sticks and did the work herself. She made sure to keep the food diverse so that even though he is stuck on 6 month old purees, he can at least enjoy nutrition and flavour.

They had two occupational therapists eventually who didn't help because their techniques were for sensory based eating. Elyot didn't have a sensory problem, he had a " what is a mouth?" problem. He had no idea what do to with his mouth. Maria would puree the foods but display the full pieces next to the plate so that Elyot at least would learn the taste and associate it with that food. If he ate pureed broccoli, there was a whole one next to the plate. He made no advances with drinking. Zero. Besides his safe space bottle he didn't learn to drink. What we discovered later was that micro preemies may have more trauma to liquids than food. Aparently oral issues are the most common issue with micro preemies but no one warned us.

Five Years Old

At the age of five he can chew his food. He can eat most types of food. He is still scared to eat but now they are working on feeding confidence, not skill training. We found a new occupational therapist who understands micro preemies and she helped us get here. The skill is now here. Drinking is from a straw still but he'll drink anything. They are working on open cups now. But we no longer worry about dehydration. Our biggest fear was that he won't be able to eat at school but he actually does. Besides having vocabulary to still advance, his communication is great. He still attends SLP sessions to learn to use more complex sentences but its just a matter of time. Physically speaking he is very strong. He loves sports and acrobatics. He does get sick often but is stronger with each year that passes.

Chapter Six
Today

It is the middle of 2021. I complete this book as we are all in worldwide isolation. Canada has had three Covid 19 surges. Everything has stopped. For me life feels the same because we had already experienced medical isolation with Elyot.

Meanwhile, my pumping did end up lasting for two years. He did end up getting RSV when he was a year old and I was in my last semester then. He got hospitalized for a week and I even graduated from the hospital room.

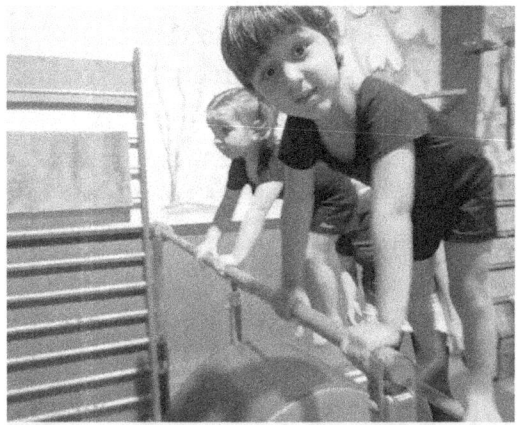

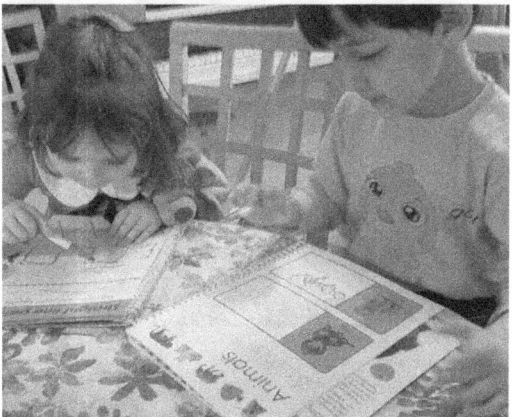

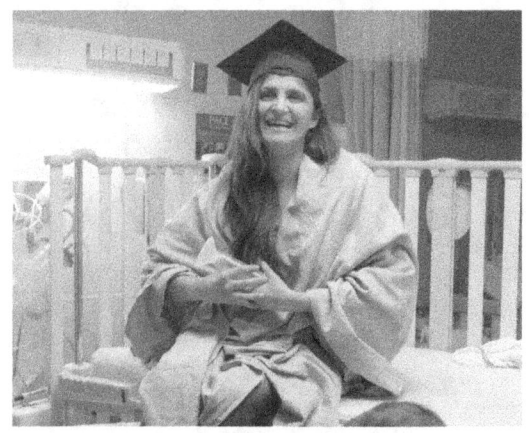

Doctors marvel at how healthy he is. He is tall and stout, a head higher than anyone his age. His favourite sport is gymnastics and like his mama he's a natural. He loves sports and joins me when I go out to unicycle. When he is ready I shall teach him to cycle as well. He loves books and is rather a nerd.

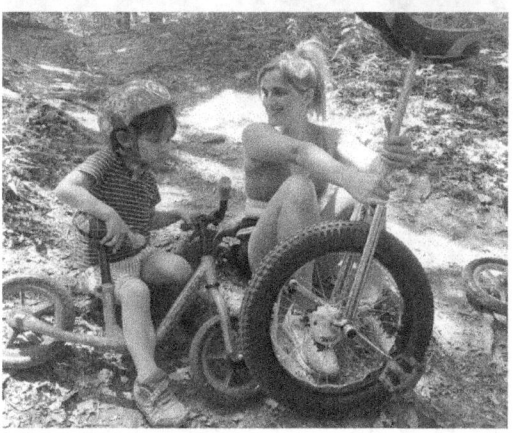

I also finally get pregnant again. I approach each week with cautious optimism, but after week 28 I start to enjoy it and look forward to my future. Notice my mask. It's the year 2020 and very scary to be pregnant. Nothing can ruin my excitement though.

She is full term and healthy. My pregnancy had no complications. I am now that other mother. I am the one for whom that bed is reserved after surgery. I am not in the long term maternity ward but only there till I can walk out. Mila latches immediately so I get to breastfeed her. Although by now I don't care how long I do it for, she is healthy. I also get a semi private room because Geoff's insurance covers it.

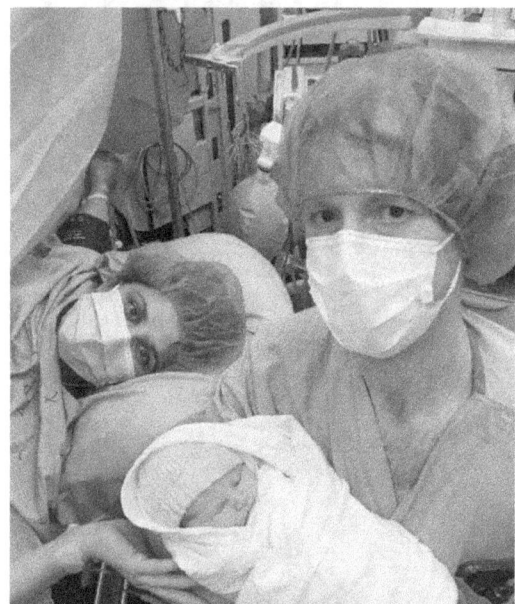

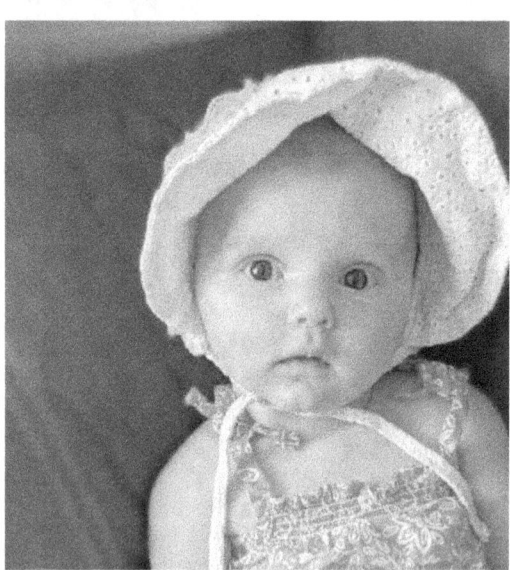

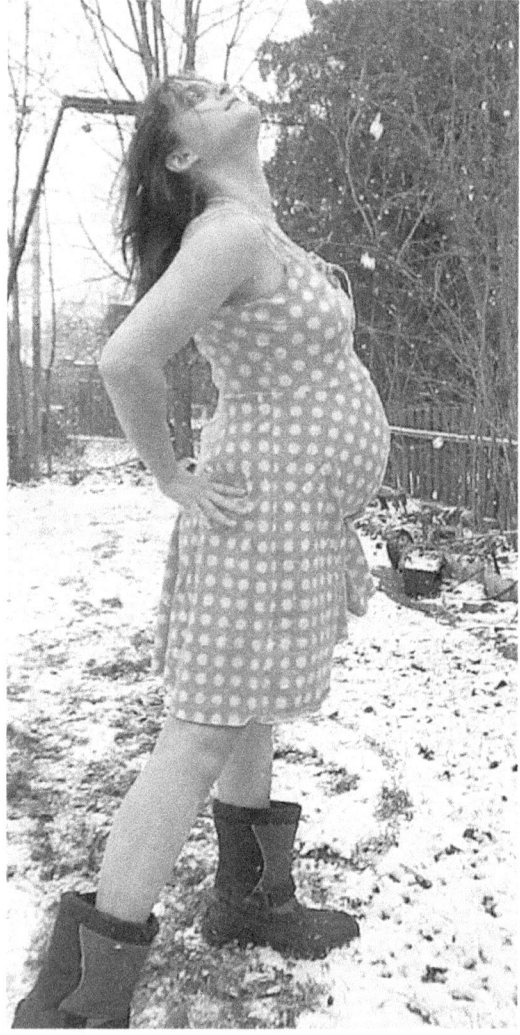

My parents have sacrificed like no one else. I wish for everyone to have the love like they do. Nothing else matters to them as much as this little boy. They spent their whole pension to pay for the expensive therapies not mentioned in the book. There is no financial support for therapy in Ontario, Canada. But Elyot benefited from a lot of early intervention. It will be a story Elyot will tell you one day if he chooses to. It's his story to tell. No one else would help us. If it wasn't for my sister or my parents I'd not be able to catch Elyot up the way I have. Thanks to them I stayed home to fill in the blanks where therapy could not. We simply did not have the money to get all that we needed. Sasha also became his therapist when she could and as a tiny village of all the Zaks we feel that by kindergarten he's doing pretty well. Thanks to Geoff being my partner in all this. These four people and no one else! You four have given him a life of happiness, agency for his own life and love.

In 2020 my parents finally move to Canada and we are all a tight unit now.

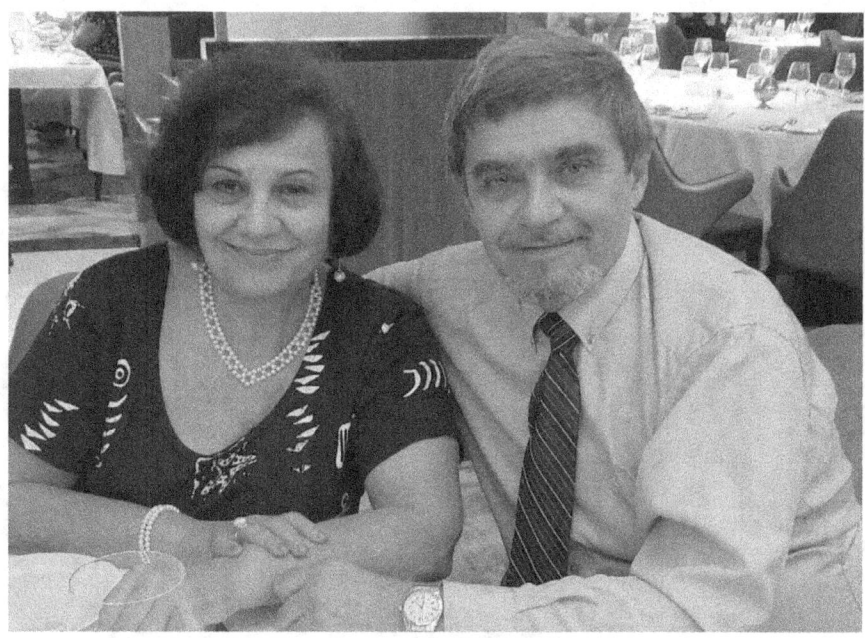

PHILIPS
17-22cm
1300
Parent

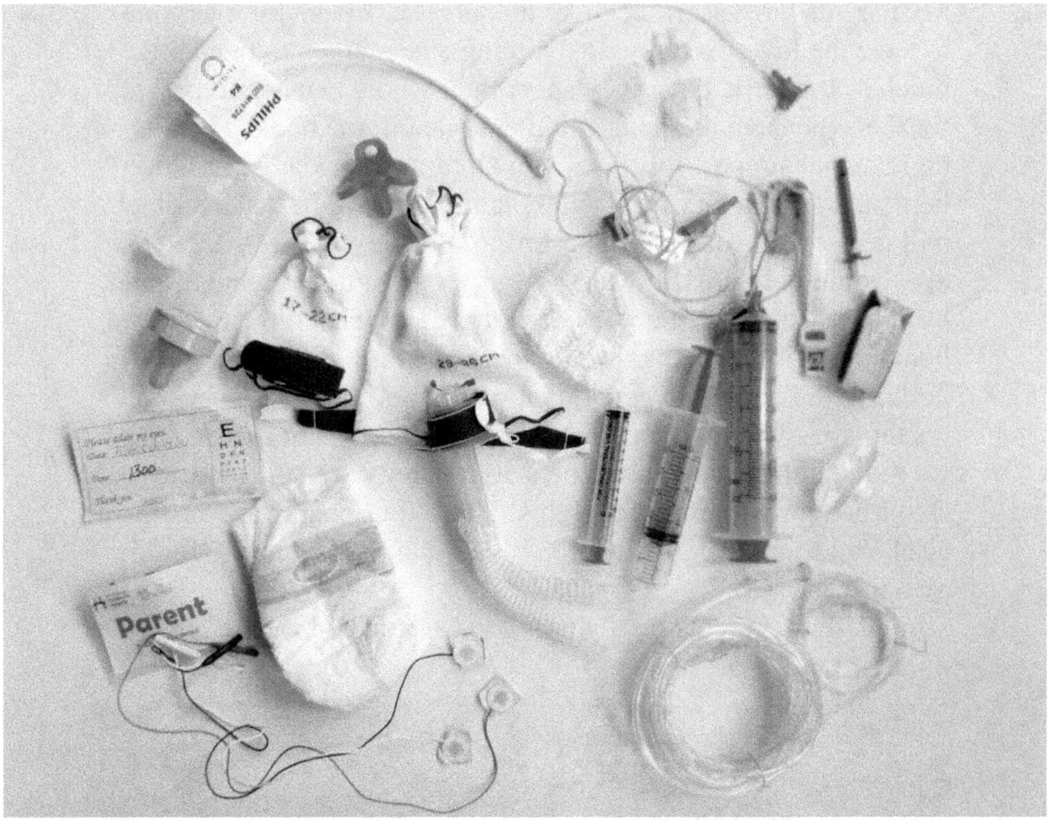

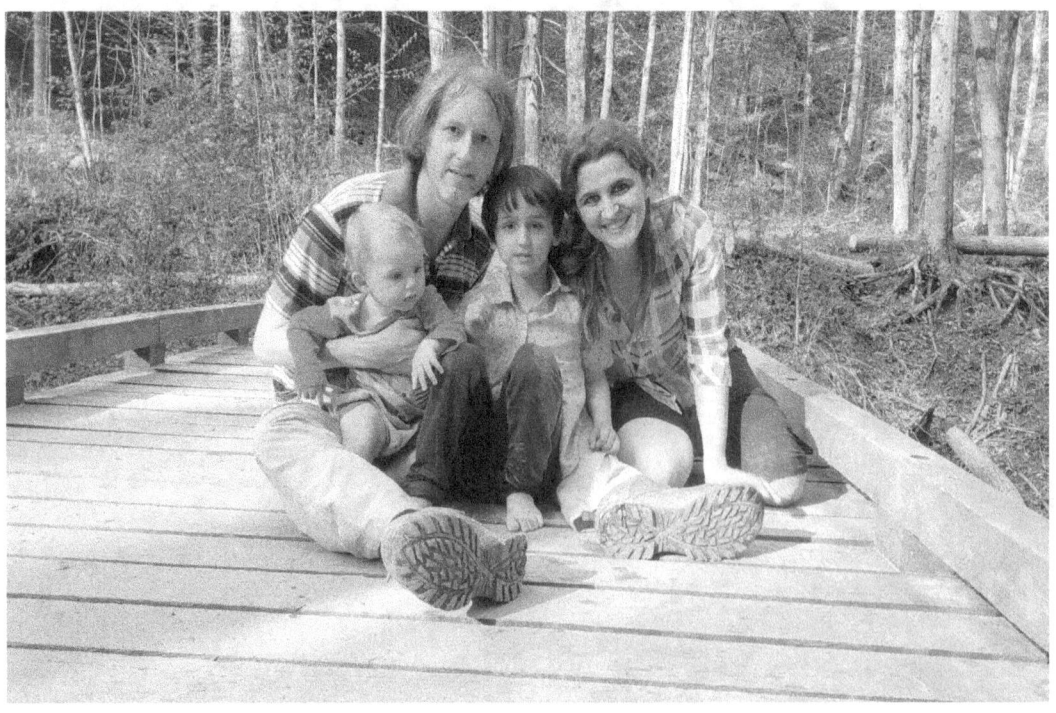

Maria and Sasha Zak are Ukrainian Canadian artists. Maria is a social worker who also works with social justice. Sasha is a therapist providing supports to children with disabilities. Together they have written for the film and theatre industry, as well as education field. Their most known work is an award winning Changezi, Dancer Among Shadows 2014 documentary.

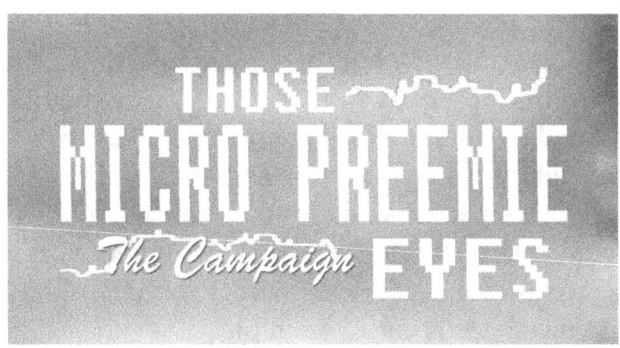

More than a book. The Zak sisters have been sharing this story to create legislative change in their communities. With each visit at a paediatric specialist or at a politician's office, a copy of this book has been shared to give a face to the issues of funding, services and hope.
Now our preemies are community activists too.

Elyot needed a lot of support but our campaign includes all other issues that are not for Elyot. We adopted all the preemies into our campaign and children with disabilities. It is an all inclusive project as you'll see.

Who gets a book?
Doctors and specialists get a book for awareness about micro preemie issues. Elyot had a severe feeding trauma and refused to touch his mouth with food, so he missed out on the milestone to learn to chew. Doctors and therapists gave us wrong strategies - mostly sensory based, and we wasted years. What he needed was oral muscle development. Doctors did not understand how being a micro preemie affected his full body. He couldn't climb, couldn't squat, had a hard time letting go of objects he picked up. I made up my own therapies but I shouldn't have to. Doctors need to know what to expect. Doctors need to know that many micro preemies will have severe colic because they cannot be burped. Many of our children will get learning disabilities and autism or physical difficulties and diagnosis. Many might even have challenges but no diagnosis. They will still need to be followed as children at risk.

A politician will get a book for legislative purposes. For funding, for community change. Parents and guardians of our children might need extra support as well. Some things we are doing in Ontario, Canada include : creating an amber alert for non verbal children and adults going missing. With local politicians we ask for more inclusive playgrounds for those using mobility devices, also to include more enrichment for children with visual impairments. We ask for sensory safe times for local shops so that people with those needs can shop in piece.

We ask for financial support for children to get the supports and therapies they need, but also for the caregivers if they have to stay home and are unable to work, to help them get through this time.

We give to schools so that they support the child holistically, but just based on a diagnosis. Also many children do not have a diagnosis but they still need the same supports.

Then we share this book with you, whoever you might be. It is a book for those who want to understand the life of a NICU family. If you are a NICU family, you are no longer alone even if your journey was a bit different. If you are someone supporting a NICU family, now you know how strong they all are.

This is the second stage of Those Eyes. The political campaign. Later we might have a follow up book on how it went and maybe updates about Elyot. Today we just want to take it a day at a time.

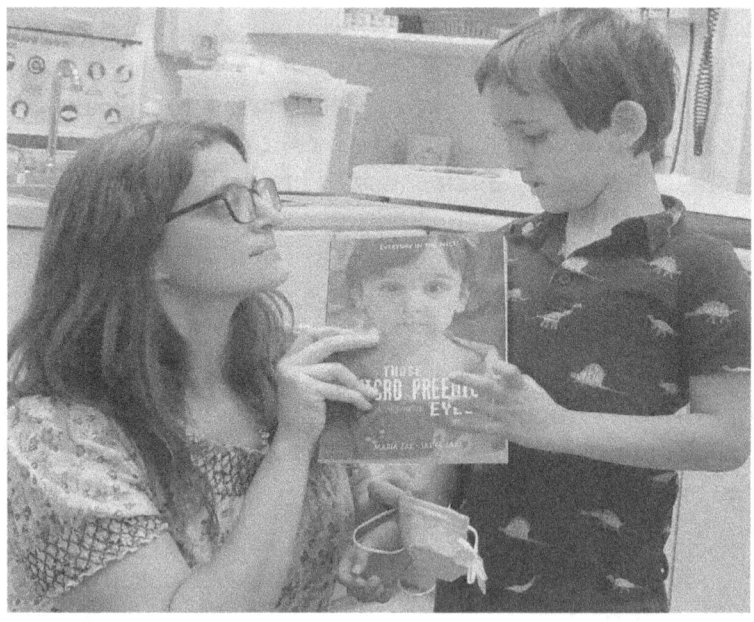

Index

Advocacy / activism
    pregnancy 3
    pumping/nursing 49, 76-80
    systemic 7, 131-138, 141-142, 146-147

Brain development
    development 59, 88, *171*
    risk assessment 27, 44, 45, 46, 50-52, 62, 93

Bunk room
    130-143, 146-147

Covid 19 references
    90, 126, 151, 166, 175

Daddy moments
    husband 63, 128
    fathering 53, 67, 68, 102, 138, 158-160, 166, 167, 170
    living far away 50, 54
    milestones 44, 45, 59, 66, 81, 101

Digestion
    51, 59, 64, 85, 105, 154
    necrotizing enterocolitis 52

Doctor
    45, 50-52, 63, 96-97

Discrimination
    at hospital 113, 131-136, 142, 146-147
    at school 56, 68, 76-80,

Equipment
    Elyot 34, 43, 44, 86, 97, 155, 129
    NICU 40, 74-75, 84-85

Eyes
    55, 59, 94

Feeding
    Bottle 146, 150, 154, 156, 157-158
    Breastfeeding 118, 128, 129, 130-143, 146-148
    Pre-oral 59, 64, 74, 85, 97, 95, 103, 105, 111

Holidays
    91, 101, 128

Low fluid
    4, 5-7, 10, 12, 14-16, 17, 23, 24-25

Lung development
    development 53, 62, 63, 86, 96-97, 105, 115-117
    equipment 85
    feeding issues 125, 138, 151
    general 50, 103
    prenatal 24
    pulling off mask 82-83

Medical interventions / therapies
    calories 105
    first interventions 50-52
    general 65, 95
    PICC 64
    prenatal steroid 24
    oxygen therapy (see Lungs)
    ROP (see Eyes)

Mental health
> *burnout* 77, 88, 97, 100, 106, 113, 115, 132, 146, 149
> *celebration* 54, 74
> *postnatal* 39
> *prenatal* 11, 14, 18, 22-23
> *pump depression* 68, 144-145

Milestones celebrations
> 59, 60, 64, 66, 74, 86, 94, 98, 101, 103, 105, 108, 111, 115, 156

Mommy moments
> *milestones* 60-61
> *mothering* 42-43, 58, 74-75, 108, 112, 115-116, 118, 154-155
> *overnight* (*see* Bunk room)

Pumping
> 21, 37, 45, 54, 89, 90
> *milk* 46-47, 98, 144-145, 155
> *pump activism* 76-80,
> *pumping everywhere* 56, 57, 68, 92, 154
> *with breastfeeding* 130-131

Regressions
> 62, 96, 129, 144-145

School
> 3-4, 12, 56, 68- 69, 77-79, 92, 175

Social worker
> 23, 68, 77, 90, 113, 132- 136, 149

Sasha's perspective
> 8, 20, 24, 25, 26-27, 34, 35, 38, 45, 50, 53, 63, 69, 84, 89, 90, 93, 100, 120, 131, 147, 163-172

Viability
> 17, 50-52, 106, 110

www.ingramcontent.com/pod-product-compliance
Lightning Source LLC
Chambersburg PA
CBHW081708100526
44590CB00022B/3704